AF823440

Official Journal of the European Stroke

Cerebrovascular Diseases

Editors-in-Chief

J. Bogousslavsky, Lausanne
M.G. Hennerici, Mannheim

Associate Editor

J.D. Easton, Providence, R.I.

Editorial Board

M.G. Bousser, Paris
L.R. Caplan, Boston, Mass.
G.J. Del Zoppo, La Jolla, Calif.
M. Fisher, Worcester, Mass.
J. van Gijn, Utrecht
P.J. Koudstaal, Rotterdam
W. Kuschinsky, Heidelberg
J.-L. Mas, Paris
J.W. Norris, Toronto
B. Norrving, Lund
S.G. Waxman, New Haven, Conn.
H. Zeumer, Hamburg

Advisory Board

H. Adams, Iowa City, Iowa
F. Aichner, Innsbruck
P. Amarenco, Paris
K. Asplund, Umeå
J.-C. Baron, Caen
R. Bonita, Auckland
N. Bornstein, Tel Aviv
G. Boysen, Copenhagen
R. Côté, Montreal
A. Dávalos, Girona
S. Davis, Parkville, Vic.
G. Devuyst, Lausanne
E. Diez-Tejedor, Madrid
G.A. Donnan, Melbourne
K. Fassbender, Mannheim
J.M. Ferro, Lisbon
N. Futrell, Salt Lake City, Utah
W. Hacke, Heidelberg
G.J. Hankey, Perth
M. Hommel, Grenoble
D. Inzitari, Florence
M. Kaps, Giessen
W. Koroshetz, Boston, Mass.
P. Langhorne, Glasgow
K.R. Lees, Glasgow
G.L. Lenzi, Rome
D. Leys, Lille
J.L. Marti-Vilalta, Barcelona
H. Mattle, Berne
J. Mau, Düsseldorf
J.P. Mohr, New York, N.Y.
E. Mori, Himeji
M.E. Moseley, Stanford, Calif.
M.A. Moskowitz, Boston, Mass.
E.B. Ringelstein, Münster
D. Russell, Oslo
W. Sandmann, Düsseldorf
J. Theron, Caen
P.J. Touboul, Paris
A. Villringer, Berlin
N.G. Wahlgren, Stockholm

KARGER

Printed in Switzerland on acid-free paper by Reinhardt Druck, Basel

Appears bimonthly: 1 volume per year (6 issues)

Cerebrovascular Diseases

Submission

Only original papers written in English are considered and should be sent to:

J. Bogousslavsky, MD
Service de Neurologie
CHUV
CH-1011 Lausanne (Switzerland)

or:

M.G. Hennerici, MD
Neurologische Klinik
Klinikum Mannheim der
Universität zu Heidelberg
Theodor-Kutzer-Ufer
D-68135 Mannheim (Germany)

Manuscripts should be submitted in quadruplicate (with four sets of illustrations of which one is an original), typewritten double-spaced on one side of the paper, with a wide margin.
At the time of the initial submission, the paper should be accompanied by the following declaration: 'The work reported in the attached paper entitled [...] has not been and is not intended to be published anywhere exept in Cerebrovascular Diseases'. The declaration should be signed by all authors.

Conditions

All manuscripts are subject to editorial review. Manuscripts are received with the explicit understanding that they are not under simultaneous consideration by any other publication. Submission of an article for publication implies the transfer of the copyright from the author to the publisher upon acceptance. Accepted papers become the permanent property of 'Cerebrovascular Diseases' and may not be reproduced by any means, in whole or in part, without the written consent of the publisher. It is the author's responsibility to obtain permission to reproduce illustrations, tables, etc. from other publications.

Arrangement

Title page: The first page of each paper should indicate the title, the authors' names, and the institute where the work was conducted. A short title for use as running head as well as the full address of the author to whom correspondence should be sent are also required.

Full address: The exact postal address complete with postal code must be given at the bottom of the title page. Please also supply phone and fax numbers, as well as your e-mail address.

Key words: For indexing purposes, a list of 3–10 key words in English is essential.

Abstract: Each paper needs an abstract of up to 10 lines.

Small type: Paragraphs which can or must be set in smaller type (case histories, test methods, etc.) should be indicated with a 'p' (petit) in the margin on the left-hand side.

Footnotes: Avoid footnotes. When essential, they are numbered consecutively and typed at the foot of the appropriate page.

Tables and illustrations: Tables and illustrations (both numbered in Arabic numerals) should be prepared on separate sheets. Tables require a heading and figures a legend, also prepared on a separate sheet. For the reproduction of illustrations, only good drawings and original photographs can be accepted; negatives or photocopies cannot be used. Due to technical reasons, figures with a screen background should not be submitted. When possible, group several illustrations on one block for reproduction (max. size 181 × 223 mm) or provide crop marks. On the back of each illustration, indicate its number, the author's name, and 'top' with a soft pencil.

Color illustrations: Up to 6 color illustrations per page can be integrated within the text at the reduced price of CHF 660.–/USD 545.00 per page. Color illustrations are reproduced at the author's expense.

References: In the text identify references by Arabic numerals [in square brackets]. Material submitted for publication but not yet accepted should be noted as 'unpublished data' and not be included in the reference list. The list of references should include only those publications which are cited in the text. Do not alphabetize; number references in the order in which they are first mentioned in the text. The surnames of the authors followed by initials should be given. There should be no punctuation other than a comma to separate the authors. Cite all authors, 'et al' is not sufficient. Abbreviate journal names according to the Index Medicus system. (Also see International Committee of Medical Journal Editors: Uniform requirements for manuscripts submitted to biomedical journals. N Engl J Med 1997;336:309–315.)

Examples
(a) Papers published in periodicals: Brenner M, Berberich R, Haass A, Schimrigk K, Pahl J: Platelet scintigraphy in cerebrovascular diseases. Eur Neurol 1989;29:197–201.
(b) Monographs: Hennerici M, Sitzer G, Weger H-D: Carotid Artery Plaques: Pathogenesis – Development – Evaluation – Treatment. Basel, Karger 1988.
(c) Edited books: Abbott NJ, Bundgaard M, Hughes CCW: Morphology of brain microvessels: A comparative approach; in Hammersen F, Messmer K (eds): Cerebral Microcirculation. Prog Appl Microcircul. Basel, Karger, 1990, vol 16, pp 1–20.

Galley proofs

Unless indicated otherwise, galley proofs are sent to the first-named author and should be returned with the least possible delay. Alterations made in galley proofs, other than the correction of printer's errors, are charged to the author. No page proofs are supplied.

Reprints

Order forms and a price list for reprints are sent with the galley proofs. Orders submitted after the issue is printed are subject to considerably higher prices.

KARGER

Fax +41 61 306 12 34
E-Mail karger@karger.ch
www.karger.com

© 2000 S. Karger AG, Basel

The Guidelines for Authors are available at:
www.karger.com/journals/ced/ced_gl.htm

Cerebrovascular Diseases

General Information

Publication data: 'Cerebrovascular Diseases' is published 6 times a year. Volume 10 with 6 issues appears in 2000.
Subscription rates: Subscriptions run for a full calendar year. Prices are given per volume.
Personal subscription:
Subscription + postage and handling
CHF 270.40 + CHF 25.90 Europe
CHF 270.40 + CHF 39.10 Overseas
USD 206.80 + USD 25.90
+ online subscription per volume:
CHF 39.– / USD 30.00
(Must be in the name of, billed to, and paid by an individual. Order must be marked 'personal subscription'.)
Institutional subscription:
Subscription + postage and handling
CHF 676.– + CHF 32.30 Europe
CHF 676.– + CHF 48.80 Overseas
USD 517.00 + USD 32.30
+ online subscription per volume:
CHF 58.– / USD 45.00
Airmail postage: CHF 36.–, USD 30.00.
(Extra per volume.)
Microforms: Please direct all enquiries and orders to: University Microfilms Inc.
300 North Zeeb Road, P.O. Box 1346
Ann Arbor, MI 48106-1346 (USA)

Subscription orders: Orders can be placed at agencies, bookstores, directly with the Publisher
S. Karger AG, P.O. Box,
CH–4009 Basel (Switzerland)
or with any of the following distributors:
Deutschland: S. Karger GmbH, Postfach
D–79095 Freiburg
France: Librairie Luginbühl
36, bd de Latour-Maubourg, F–75007 Paris
Great Britain, Ireland: S. Karger Publishers
58 Grove Hill Road
Tunbridge Wells, Kent TN1 1SP
USA: S. Karger Publishers, Inc.
26 West Avon Road, P.O. Box 529
Farmington, CT 06085
India, Bangladesh, Sri Lanka:
S. Karger India Subscription Agency
B–5/132 Safdarjung Enclave
New Delhi 110029
Japan: Katakura Libri, Inc.
2F, Marushima Bldg, 4-6-17, Yushima,
Bunkyo-ku, Tokyo 113-0034
Change of address: Both old and new address should be sent to the subscription source.
Single issues and back volumes: Information can be obtained through the Publisher.

Advertising: Correspondence and rate requests should be addressed to the Publisher.
Bibliographic indices: This journal is regularly listed in bibliographic services, including *Current Contents*® and Index Medicus/MEDLINE.
Copying: This journal has been registered with the Copyright Clearance Center (CCC), as indicated by the code appearing on the first page of each article.
For readers in the US, this code signals consent for copying of articles for personal or internal use, or for the personal or internal use of specific clients, provided that the stated fee is paid per copy directly to
Copyright Clearance Center Inc.
222 Rosewood Drive
Danvers, MA 01923 (USA)
A copy of the first page of the article must accompany payment. Consent does not extend to copying for general distribution, for promotion, for creating new works, or for resale. In these cases, specific written permission must be obtained from the copyright owner,
S. Karger AG,
P.O. Box, CH–4009 Basel (Switzerland).

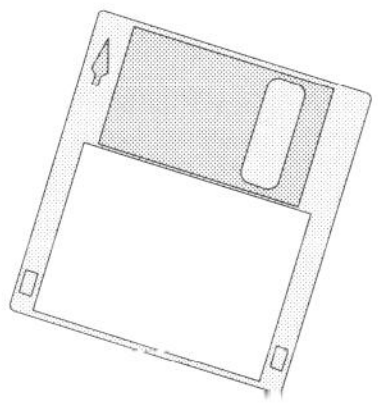

Disk Submission

A **comprehensive version** of these guidelines for the **submission of manuscripts and illustrations on disk** can be accessed online under **www.karger.com/journals/disksub.htm** or requested as a leaflet from the editorial department.

Please follow the general rules on style and arrangement in the **'Guidelines for Authors'** of the journal. Submit a **double-spaced printout** of your manuscript matching the file on disk exactly.

Technical Information

Store only data pertinent to this manuscript. Include your fonts (screen and printer fonts for Macintosh).
For a **text only** manuscript, use a 3.5 inch disk.
For **text and illustrations,** use 3.5 or 5.25 Magneto Optical Disc; CD-ROM (DOS or hybrid); iomage Zip/DOS (100 MB), or 44 MB, 88 MB or 200 MB SyQuest. Compress extensive data using ZIP format.

Data Description

Label your disk with the **title of the journal or book** for which it is submitted; a **short version** of the paper's title; your **name,** postal and e-mail address, fax and phone number; **hard and software** used, including the version; and the **complete list of the file names.** File names consist of eight characters before the dot identifying the file and three characters after the dot identifying the application.

Text and Format

The **preferred word-processing package is MS-Word.** Other commonly used PC text programs and ASCII formats are accepted.
Update your data when you revise subsequent to the reviewer's or editor's decision and mark revisions clearly. Manuscripts accepted for publication are subject to **copy editing:** changes and/or questions will be marked in the manuscript, which will be returned to you with your disk and the galley proofs for checking.
Enter your text continuously flush left. Do not use any layout functions. Do not split words at the end of a line. **Do not use indentations.** Use a blank line before and a hard return at the end of paragraphs.
Arrange headings flush left. Insert only **one space after punctuation marks.** Insert Greek letters, mathematical symbols etc. with your word-processing program. Use **boldface and italics** as well as sub- and superscript where appropriate.
Tables are part of the text and should be placed at the end of the text file. Separate the individual parts of a table by lines. Use the tabulator instead of spaces. Format operation data on one line in the same column. **Legends to illustrations are part of the text** and should also be listed at the end of the text file.

Illustrations

Store illustrations as separate files: do not integrate them in your text. Export **line drawings/vector graphics** as TIF, EPS or WMF format. Use Photoshop for processing and retouching **scanned halftone images.** Save the original scan and the processed version. Export **black and white or color images** as TIF or EPS format in their anticipated size in print.
For detailed information on how to submit illustration data on disk please consult the leaflet or **www.karger.com/journals/disksub.htm.**

© 2000 S. Karger AG, Basel

Fax + 41 61 306 12 34
E-Mail karger@karger.ch
www.karger.com

The Journal Home Page is available at:
www.karger.com/journals/ced

Karger Journals in . . .

. . . Neuroscience

Biological Signals and Receptors An international forum for experimental research on the production, transmission, processing, recognition and effect of biological signals	**Brain, Behavior and Evolution** Focuses on morphological, physiological and behavioral studies of vertebrate and invertebrate nervous systems and their evolution	**Cerebrovascular Diseases** Featuring clinical research advances in stroke and cerebrovascular diseases as well as the latest information on diagnostic testing and therapeutics	**Dementia and Geriatric Cognitive Disorders** Examines the neural bases of cognitive dysfunction, concentrating on Alzheimer's, Parkinson's, and other neurodegenerative diseases
Developmental Neuroscience Featuring multidisciplinary neuroscience papers covering all stages of invertebrate, vertebrate and human development	**European Neurology** Covering neuropathological, biochemical, electrophysiological and clinical aspects of diseases of the nervous system and muscles	**Neuroendocrinology** A frequently cited source of original data on the multiple complex interactions between the endocrine and nervous systems throughout the body	**Neuroepidemiology** Concerned with descriptive, analytical and experimental aspects of neurologic disease
NeuroImmunoModulation Encompassing both basic and clinical research, this journal investigates the complex interactions of the nervous and immune systems	**Neuropsychobiology** A complete record of strategies and methodologies employed in the biological approach to mental disorders	**Pediatric Neurosurgery** New information and observations in pediatric neurosurgery and the allied fields of neuroradiology and neuropathology	**Stereotactic and Functional Neurosurgery** Featuring state-of-the-art clinical and technical developments to meet the information needs of both investigators and clinicians

Write, fax or e-mail for a free sample copy!

KARGER

S. Karger AG
P.O. Box, CH–4009 Basel
(Switzerland)
Tel. +41 61 306 11 11
Fax +41 61 306 12 34
E-mail karger@karger.com

S. Karger Publishers, Inc.
26 West Avon Road
P.O. Box 529
Farmington, CT 06085 (USA)
Toll free: 1-800-828-5479
Fax +1 860 675-7302

For easy ordering or further information on Karger publications log on to:
www.karger.com

KI 00440

Cerebrovascular
Diseases

5th Meeting of the European Society of Neurosonology and Cerebral Hemodynamics

Graz, Austria, May 21–23, 2000

Abstracts

Guest Editors
K. Niederkorn, Graz
S. Horner, Graz
D. Russell, Oslo

KARGER

Basel · Freiburg · Paris · London · New York ·
New Delhi · Bangkok · Singapore · Tokyo · Sydney

S. Karger
Medical and Scientific Publishers
Basel · Freiburg · Paris · London
New York · New Delhi · Bangkok
Singapore · Tokyo · Sydney

Drug Dosage
The authors and the publisher have exerted every effort to ensure that drug selection and dosage set forth in this text are in accord with current recommendations and practice at the time of publication. However, in view of ongoing research, changes in government regulations, and the constant flow of information relating to drug therapy and drug reactions, the reader is urged to check the package insert for each drug for any change in indications and dosage and for added warnings and precautions. This is particularly important when the recommended agent is a new and/or infrequently employed drug.

All rights reserved.
No part of this publication may be translated into other languages, reproduced or utilized in any form or by any means, electronic or mechanical, including photocopying, recording, microcopying, or by any information storage and retrieval system, without permission in writing from the publisher or, in the case of photocopying, direct payment of a specified fee to the Copyright Clearance Center (see 'General Information').

© Copyright 2000 by S. Karger AG,
P.O. Box, CH–4009 Basel (Switzerland)
Printed in Austria by
Medienfabrik Graz, Steiermärkische Landesdruckerei GmbH
ISBN 3–8055–7109–7

KARGER

Fax+ 41 61 306 12 34
E-Mail karger@karger.ch
www.karger.com

WELCOME TO GRAZ

On behalf of the Organizing Committee we are very pleased to announce that the 5th Meeting of the European Society of Neurosonology and Cerebral Hemodynamics will be held in Graz, May 21st – 23rd 2000, immediately preceeding the 9th European Stroke Conference, Vienna, May 24th–27th.
Neurosonology and its use in the acute setting of the Stroke Unit will be covered as well as the latest developments in the field of echocontrast agents, embolus detection, IMT measurement and functional and neurointerventional aspects of TCD.
Advanced tutorials on TCD Embolus Monitoring and Transcranial Colour Duplex Sonography including the application of contrast agents will be held.

Graz, Austria's "Queen of Hearts" was described as follows:
"Although with a quarter of a million inhabitants it`s the second largest city in Austria, it is still homely, green and fairly provincial, say some. The city has culture, three universities and a lively bar scene, say others. In fact, both are right:
Graz is bourgeois and cosmopolitan, idyllic and full of life, traditional and avant-garde.

The meeting will be held in the Grazer Kongreß Convention Center which combines old world charme with modern equipment and up-to-date presentation and exhibition facilities.
We will do our best to progress the meeting not only on a high scientific level but also, with the help of traditional Austrian hospitality, as a social event worth to remember.

Prof. Kurt Niederkorn	Dr. Susanna Horner
Congress Chairman	Congress Secretary

This meeting is co-sponsored by the Neurosonology Research Group of the World Federation of Neurology
The Austrian Society of Neuroimaging

COMMITTEES

European Society of Neurosonology and Cerebral Hemodynamics

President: D. Russell, Norway
Secretary: J. Klingelhöfer, Germany
Treasurer: E. Bartels, Germany

Executive Committee Members:

R. Ackerstaff, The Netherlands
D. Grossett, UK
K. Niederkorn, Austria
E. B. Ringelstein, Germany
E. Zanette, Italy

Local Organizing Committee:

K. Niederkorn, *Chairman*
S. Horner, *Secretary*
D. Russell, *Society President*

M. Augustin
R. Fischer
G. Grinschgl
B. Pieberl
T. Schober

CORE SCIENTIFIC COMMITTEE

R. Aaslid, USA
R.G. Ackerstaff, The Netherlands
F. Aichner, Austria
E. Bartels, Germany
N. Bornstein, Israel
J. M. de Bray, France
L. Csiba, Hungary
V. Demarin, Croatia
F. Fazekas, Austria
D. Grosset, UK
M. Hennerici, Germany
M. Kaps, Germany
J. Klingelhöfer, Germany
H. Markus, UK
K. Niederkorn, Austria
V. Oliveira, Portugal
G. M. von Reutern, Germany
E. B. Ringelstein, Germany
D. Russell, Norway
M. Siebler, Germany
M. Sturzenegger, Switzerland
P. Traubner, Slovakia
E.M. Zanette, Italy

INTERNATIONAL SCIENTIFIC COMMITTEE

G. Acerbi, Italy
G.P. Anzola, Italy
P. Arbeille, France
V. I. Babikian, USA
P. Bartenstein, Germany
R. Brucher, Germany
A. Dahl, Norway
D. Droste, Germany
D. H. Evans, UK
C. Fieschi, Italy
R. Frackowiak, UK
H. Furuhata, Japan
D. Georgiadis, Germany
C. A. Giller, USA
D. Giobbe, Italy
C. R. Gomez, USA
B. Griewing, Germany
A. Hetzel, Germany
S. Horner, Austria
D. G. Iacopino, Italy
Z. Kalibutowska, Poland
P. Kalvach, Czech Republic
G. Ladurner, Austria
P. Limoni, Italy
M. Mattle, Switzerland
S. Meairs, Germany
G. Meneghetti, Italy
D.W. Newell, USA
S. C. Nicholls, USA
G. A. Ottonello, Italy
K. Paulat, Germany
F. Ries, Germany
S.-J. Ryu, Taiwan
P. E. Roland, Sweden
T.V. Schroeder, Denmark
M. del Sette, Italy
V. A. Shakhnovich, Russia
M. Sloan, USA
M. P. Spencer, USA
D. A. Stump, USA
C. H. Tegeler, USA
E. Titianova, Bulgaria
J. P. Touboul, France
T. Totaro, Italy
M. Visocchi, Italy
C. Weiller, Germany
C. Werner, Germany
B. Widder, Germany
B. Zvan, Slovenia

GENERAL INFORMATION

CONGRESS VENUE

Grazer Congress Convention Center,
Schmiedgasse 2, A-8010 Graz, Austria
Tel.: ++43/316/8049 0
Fax: ++43/316/82 64 67
E-Mail: office@gcongress.com

COMMERCIAL EXHIBITION:

organized by Grazer Congress Convention Center
Mrs. Eva Puchwein

SOCIAL EVENTS:

Welcome Reception by the Major of the City of Graz, Alfred Stingl, Congress Venue, Sunday, May 21, 7.00 p.m.

Reception by the Governor of Styria, Mrs. Waltraud Klasnic, Graz Burg, Monday, May 22, 8.00 p.m.

Sightseeing Tour through old Graz, Monday, May 22, 10.00 a.m.–12.30 p.m.

LANGUAGE

The official language of the congress is English.

CONGRESS FEE

ATS 3200, (EUR 232,60)

TUTORIAL

ATS 1200,– (EUR 87,20)

Attendants registered with the 9th European Stroke Conference, Vienna, May 24th-27th, 2000 are entitled to ATS 500,– discount on registration fees (not Tutorial) by presenting a copy of the registration.

MEANS OF PAYMENT

1. **Eurocheque** (ATS 2.500,– EUR 181,69 maximum per cheque) or bankers cheque payable to the order of: "Neurosonology 2000".
2. **Bank transfer** to the Hypo Bank Graz, account no.: 20241072674, Bank code 56000 **without charges for the beneficiary.**
3. **Credit card:** the following credit cards will be accepted: Eurocard/Mastercard, Visa

ACCOMPANYING PERSONS

FREE OF CHARGE

ABSTRACTS

All abstracts accepted are published in a supplement of Cerebrovascular Diseases.

HOTEL RESERVATION:

City Tourist Office Graz
Mrs. Gudrun Jäger
P.O.Box 183, Kaiserfeldgasse 15, A-8010 Graz
Tel.: ++43/316/80 75 -Ext. 59-62
Fax: ++43/316/80 75 55
e-mail: gj@graztourismus.at

CONGRESS SECRETARIAT:

Prof. Kurt Niederkorn
Dept. of Neurology
Karl-Franzens-University of Graz
Auenbruggerplatz 22
A-8036 Graz, Austria
Tel.: ++43/316/31-82-08
Fax: ++43/316/31-82-08/24
E-Mail: kurt.niederkorn@kfunigraz.ac.at

or
nsrg@sime.com

Website:
http:/www.kfunigraz.ac.at/neuwww/esnch2000.html

From May 20,
Grazer Congress Convention Center,
Schmiedgasse 2, A-8010 Graz, Austria
Tel.: ++43/316/8049-82 and ++43/664/49-47-094
Fax: ++43/316/82 64 67
E-Mail: office@gcongress.com

Opening hours of the Congress Secretariat and Registration Desk:

Saturday, May 20,	15.00 – 19.00
Sunday, May 21,	07.30 – 19.00
Monday, May 22,	07.30 – 19.00
Tuesday, May 22,	07.30 – 16.00

Technical Information

Invited Lectures:

15 minutes speaking time plus 5 minutes discussion

Oral Presentations:

8 minutes speaking time plus 2 minutes discussion

Slide Projection:

Single and double projection (35 mm) is available in all lecture halls.

Video Projection (SVHS,VHS) and Data Projection (Windows 95,98,NT; Power Point Presentations) is available in the hall Steiermarksaal.

Posters (poster walls measure 97x250 cm) can be mounted on Monday, May 22, starting at 08.00 a.m. and must be taken down on Tuesday, May 23, in the afternoon.

FINAL SCIENTIFIC PROGRAM

TUTORIALS

TUTORIAL I

Sunday, May 21, 9.00 a.m.–12.30 p.m,
Hall: Ausstellungshalle

TCD EMBOLUS MONITORING
Faculty: H. Markus, D. Georgiadis, S. Horner

The tutorial will consist of 2 parts of 90 minutes each separated by a 30 minutes break.

In the first part lectures will cover the issues of spontaneous embolization to the brain in various conditions like carotid stenosis, atrial fibrillation, valvular heart disease as well as the diagnosis paradoxical embolism via right-to-left shunts. Technical and clinical aspects will be addressed alike.

The second 90 minutes are mainly devoted to detailed case presentations.

TUTORIAL II

TRANSCRANIAL COLOUR DUPLEX SONOGRAPHY
(including application of contrast agents)

Sunday, May 21, 9.00 a.m.–12.30 p.m, Hall: K 1–2

Faculty: G.M. von Reutern, E. Bartels, M. Goertler

The tutorial will consist of 2 parts of 90 minutes each separated by a 30 minutes break.

In the first part lectures will cover technical aspects including the use of contrast agents, clinical results and limitations of the methods in the anterior and posterior intracranial circulation as well as the investigation of brain parenchymal abnormalities.

The second part is a hands-on session, including a detailed clinical demonstration.

SCIENTIFIC SESSIONS

Sunday, May 21, 2000, Hall: Steiermarksaal

13.45–14.00	Opening
14.00–16.00	**Session I:** Embolus Detection – Technical Aspects
16.30–18.30	**Session II:** Embolus Detection – Clinical Aspects

Monday, May 22, 2000, Hall: Steiermarksaal

08.30–10.30	**Session III:** IMT Measurement and Primary Stroke Prevention
11.00–13.00	**Session IV:** Neurosurgical and Neurointerventional Aspects of Neurosonology
14.00–16.00	**Session V:** Poster Session (Hall: Ausstellungssaal and K 1–2)
16.30–18.30	**Session VI:** Autoregulation Testing and Functional Aspects of TCD

Special Symposia, Hall: Blauer Salon

08.30 –09.30	Neuronavigation
09.30–11.00	Noninvasive Monitoring of Cerebral Function

Tuesday, May 23, 2000, Hall: Steiermarksaal

08.30–10.30	**Session VII:** Echocontrast Agents – Latest Developments
11.00–13.00	**Session VIII:** Work in Progress and Future Aspects of Neurosonology
14.00–16.00	**Session IX:** Neurosonology and Neuroimaging in Acute Stroke
16.00	Adjourn

KARGER
Fax + 41 61 306 12 34
E-Mail karger@karger.ch
www.karger.com

© 2000 S. Karger AG, Basel

Sunday, May 21, 2000

Opening: 13.45–14.00

Session I: 14.00 – 16.00

EMBOLUS DETECTION – TECHNICAL ASPECTS

Chairmen: R. BRUCHER, D. EVANS

Invited Speakers:

14.00 D. RUSSELL
Recent Advances in Embolus Detection and Differentiation

14.20 H. MARKUS
Automatic Detection of Cerebral Emboli

14.40 *Automated Emboli Identification: Detection Using a Combination of Time and Frequency Domain*
1 *Information*
L. Fan, D. H. Evans, A. R. Naylor (UK)

14.50 *A New Method for Automatic Differentiation between Cerebral Emboli and Artefacts*
2 R.Brucher, D.Russell (Germany, Norway)

15.00 *Comparison of a New On-Line Automated Embolic*
3 *Signal Detection Algorithm with a Panel of Human Experts*
M.Cullinane, G.Reid, R.Ackerstaff, V.Babikian,
D.Droste, M.Siebler, L.Valton. D.G Grosset, H.S Markus (UK)

15.10 *Evaluation of a New On Line Automated Embolic Signal Detection Algorithm*
4 R. Dittrich, M. Cullinane, G. Reid, Z. Kaposzta, H. S. Markus (UK)

15.20 *The Matching Pursuit has the Potential to Characterize the Nature – Gaseous or Solid – of Microembolic*
5 *Signals by Transcranial Doppler Ultrasound. The Walvelet Study Group.*
G.Devuyst, J.M.Vesin, G.de Freitas, N.Cals, N.Afsar, J. Rohr-le-Floch, R.Sztatjzel, J.Serena, C.Molina, M. Ossemann, M.Ritter, D.Droste, E.B Ringelstein, P.A.Despland, J. Bogousslavsky (Switzerland, Germany)

15.30 *In Vitro Evaluation of the Mechanism for "Tail Signs" Associated with Microembolic Signals*
6 E. Furui, K. Hanzawa, T. Nakajima, N. Fukuhara, K. Komai, M.Yamada (Japan)

15.40 *Microembolus Tracking with Power M-Mode Transcranial Doppler Ultrasound and Simultaneous Single*
7 *Gate Spectrogram*
M.A.Moehring (Germany)

15.50 *Postembolic Spectral Patterns of Microembolic Signals*
8 F. Uhlmann, W. J. Schulte-Mattler, D. Georgiadis (Germany)

Session II: 16.30–18.30

EMBOLUS DETECTION – CLINICAL ASPECTS

Chairmen: D. RUSSELL, M. SIEBLER

Invited Speakers:

16.30 R. G. ACKERSTAFF
Embolus Detection in Surgical and Interventional Procedures of the Carotid Arteries

16.50 D. DROSTE
Clinical Relevance of Spontaneous Carotid Emboli

17.10 *Asymptomatic Carotid Emboli Study (ACES)*
9 H.Markus, M.Cullinane (UK)

17.20 *Asymptomatic Stenosis Embolus Detection (ASED) Study*
10 A.Harris, B.Chambers, J.Stok, C.Levi, C.Bladin, G.Donnan (Australia)

17.30 *Cerebral Microembolism Corresponds to Antiplatelet Medication in Patients with Symptomatic Arterial*
11 *Stenosis*
S. Krueger, T. Blaser, C. W. Wallesch, M. Goertler, (Germany)

17.40 *Doppler Microembolic Signals During Cardiac Surgery*
12 D.Georgiadis, R.Stets, A.Schorcht, A.Hempel, F.Uhlmann, G.Fischer, R.E. Silber, H.R.Zerkowski, S.Zierz (Germany)

17.50 *Antiplatelets Reduced Non-Gaseous Hits in Patients with Mechanical Valve*
13 K.Hanzawa, E.Furui, S.Namura, H.Moro, M.Kitamura, T.Nakajima, N.Fukuhara, J-I.Hayashi, H.Naritomi (Japan)

18.00 *Patent Foramen Ovale and Obstructive Apnea Syndrome*
14 M. Del Sette, S.Angeli, F.Ferrillo, M.Beelke, L.Nobili, S.Pretta, C.Gandolfo (Italy)

18.10 *GPIIb/IIIa Platelet Receptor Antagonists in Acute Ischemic Stroke*
15 M.Siebler, U.Junghans, R.Seitz (Germany)

18.20 *S-Nitrosoglutathione, a Platelet Specific Nitric Oxide Donor, and L-Arginine Reduce Embolisation post*
16 *Carotid Endarterectomy*
Z.Kaposzta, P.A.Baskerville, S.C.A.Fraser, D.Madge, J.F.Martin, HS.Markus, (UK)

Monday, May 22, 2000

SPECIAL SYMPOSIA (Hall: Blauer Salon)

NEURONAVIGATION, 8.30–9.30

Chairman: M. SIEBLER

Faculty: M. SIEBLER, A. KRONE

M. SIEBLER
Ultrasound Applications in Navigation: an Introduction

A. KRONE
Neuronavigation: Intraoperative Ultrasound during Neurosurgery

NONINVASIVE MONITORING OF CEREBRAL FUNCTION, 9.30–11.00

Chairman: D. RUSSELL

Faculty: D. RUSSELL, R. BRUCHER, K. PAULAT

This special symposium will provide a state of the art-update regarding how cerebral function may now be monitored non-invasively and how this information can help in patient management. The three most important parameters in this regard are:

1. Solid or Gaseous Cerebral Embolization
2. Blood Flow in the Major Intracranial Arteries
3. Intracranial Pressure and Compliance

The Symposium will demonstrate how recent research has greatly improved the possibility to non-invasively assess these parameters. Basic principles will be discussed and clinical examples provided.

Session III: 8.30–10.30

IMT MEASUREMENTS AND PRIMARY STROKE PREVENTION

Chairmen: V. DEMARIN, N. BORNSTEIN

Invited Speakers:

08.30	J. KLINGELHÖFER *Risk Factor Correlations*
08.50	M. SITZER *Chlamydia Pneumoniae Infection and Early Asymptomatic Carotid Atherosclerosis*
09.10 **17**	*Can Intima-Media Thickness Predict Risk of Stroke in Patients with Acute Myocardial Infarction* V.Oliveira, A.Pedro, P.Batista, F.Soares (Portugal)
09.20 **18**	*Reduced Progression of Early Atherosclerosis Following Antibiotic Therapy after Ischemic Stroke and Chlamydia Pneumoniae Seropositivity* D. Sander, K. Winbeck, J. Klingelhöfer, B. Heyse, J.Schwarze, B. Conrad (Germany)

09.30 *Elevated C-Reactive Protein is Associated with an Increased Early Atherosclerosis*
19 K. Winbeck, Ch. Kulka, B. Heyse, J. Klingelhöfer, B. Conrad, D. Sander (Germany)

09.40 *Increased Carotid Artery Intima-Media Thickness in U.K. African Caribbeans*
20 Z. Kaposzta, M. Cullinane, R. Dittrich, C. Wolfe, H. S. Markus (UK)

09.50 *Intima-Media Thickness and Ambulatory Blood Pressure Monitoring in Hypertensive Patients*
21 C.Barone, F.Nobili, N.R.Musso, V. De Iorgi, F. Copello, G.Lotti, G.Rodriguez (Italy)

10.00 *Aging Dependent Decrease in the Cerebral Autoregulation after Adrenergic Stimulation by Hand-Grip*
22 S.Castellani, I.Carobbi, N.Boni, V.Corsoni, F.Lavorini, C.Zeloni, F.Battaglia, G.F.Gensini, G.Masotti (Italy)

10.10. *Impaired Cerebrovascular Reactivity Predicts Stroke and TIA Risk in Carotid Artery Disease;*
23 *A Prospective Study*
M.Cullinane, H.S.Markus (UK)

10.20 *Detection of Circle of Willis Collaterals: MRA Compared to Transcranial Duplex Scanning*
24 A. W. J.Hoksbergen, D. A.Legemate, C.B.L.M, Majoie, F. J. H. Hulsmans (The Netherlands)

Session IV: 11.00 – 13.00

NEUROSURGICAL AND NEUROINTERVENTIONAL ASPECTS OF NEUROSONOLOGY

Chairmen: P. LIMONI, A. SHAKHNOVICH

Invited Speakers:

11.00 E. KLEIN
The Potential of Neurointervention in Acute Ischemic Stroke and SAH

11.20 M. VISOCCHI
Neurosonology and Neuromodulation of CBF by Electrical Stimulation

11.40 *Intraoperative Transcranial Doppler Monitoring and the Prediction of Stroke from Carotid Endarterectomy*
25 R. G. A. Ackerstaff, M. P. Spencer, C. J. W. van der Vlasakker, F. L. Moll, F. E. E. Vermeulen, A. Algra, G. M. Moons (The Netherlands, USA)

11.50 *Are Carotid Stents a Source of Microemboli Late After Deployment?*
26 B.Censori, T.Partziguian, L.Casto, M.Camerlingo, A.Mamoli (Italy)

12.00 *The Risk Factors of Severe Brain Ischemia (SBI) during Carotid Endarterectomy (CE) and ICA Clamping*
27 V. A. Shakhnovich, V. A. Lazarev, G. E. Mitroshin, M. V. Churilov, D. Y. Usachev, A. A. Shmigelsky, A. Y. Lubnin (Russia)

12.10 *Duplex Ultrasound in Neuronavigation of Deep-Seated Cavernomas*
28 R. Stendel, A. Abo Al Hassan, M. Brock (Germany)

12.20 *Feeding Artery Detection and Monitoring of Basal Artery Hemodynamics with Color-Duplex-Sonography*
29 *During Surgery of Arteriovenous Angiomas*
M. Woydt, A. Krone, J. Meixensberger, K. Roosen (Germany)

12.30 *Autoregulation Testing for Cerebral Arteriovenous Malformation (AVM) Surgery*
30 A. L. Krivoshapkin, E. G. Melidy, V. V. Fonin, P. A. Semin, V. V. Kanygin (Russia)

12.40 *Multiparameter Sensors and Microdialysis Monitoring during Aneurysm Surgery: Predictive Value for*
31 *Infarction*
R. Kett-White, P. J. Hutchinson, P Al-Rawi, A.Gupta, P.J Kirkpatrick (UK)

12.50 *Investigation of Transcranial Doppler (TCD) Power Output for Potentiation of Tissue Plasminogen*
32 *Activator (tPA) Therapy in Stroke*
M. A. Moehring, A. H.Voie, M. P. Spencer, D. W. Amory, AV. Alexandrov (USA)

13.30 **General Meeting of the European Society of Neurosonology and Cerebral Hemodynamics, Hall: Steiermarksaal**

Session VI: 16.30 – 18.30

AUTOREGULATION TESTING AND FUNCTIONAL ASPECTS OF TCD

Chairmen: E. B. RINGELSTEIN, K. PAULAT

Invited Speakers:

16.30 E.B. RINGELSTEIN
Functional TCD for Brain Research

16.50 L. CSIBA
New Aspects of TCD Measurements in High Stroke Risk Populations

17.10 *Vasomotor Reactivity of Anterior Cerebral Artery in Patients with Carotid Occlusive Disease*
33 N. M. Bornstein, A.Y.Gur, T.Nissel, S.Lorenz (Israel)

17.20 *Time Delay as Parameter for Cerebrovascular Reactivity in Patients with Severe Carotid Stenosis*
34 A. Hetzel, G. Guschlbauer (Germany)

17.30 *Introduction of a Reading Paradigm for Neurovascular Coupling and Mobilie f-TCD*
35 B. Rosengarten, M. Kaps (Germany)

17.40 *TCD Changes in Patients with Autonomic Neuropathy*
36 B. Zvan, M. Zaletel, T. Pogacnik (Slovenia)

17.50 *Transcranial Doppler Monitoring during Head-down Tilt: A Tool to Investigate Non-Sympathetic Cerebral*
37 *Autoregulatory Pathway*
D. Bosone, V. Ozturk, S. Roatta, A. Cavallini, P. Tosi, G. Micieli (Italy, Turky)

18.00 *Cerebral Hemodynamics During Vasovagal Syncope*
38 B. J. Carey, P. J. Eames, R. P. Panerai, J. F. Potter (UK)

18.10 *Cerebral Blood Flow Velocity (CBFV) during Upright Tilt in Chronic Fatigue Syndrom (CFS)*
39 A. Razumovsky, K. DeBusk, H.Calkins, S. Snader, P. Vyas, D. Hanley, P. C. Rowe (USA)

18.20 *B- and M-Waves in Various Types of Headache*
40 U. Sliwka, S. Harscher, R. V. Schayck, C. C. Eschenfelder, C.Weiller (Germany)

Tuesday, May 23, 2000

Session VII: 8.30–10.30

ECHOCONTRAST AGENTS – LATEST DEVELOPMENTS

Chairpersons: E. BARTELS, J.M. DE BRAY

Invited Speakers:

08.30 D. NABAVI
The Use of Echocontrast Agents in Clinical Practice

08.50 G. SEIDEL
Present State and Potentials of Harmonic Imaging

09.10 *Harmonic Imaging of the Basal Cerebral Arteries*
41 S. Horner, M. Augustin, G. Bone, E. Klein, R. Schmidt, T. Schober, K. Niederkorn (Austria)

09.20 *Comparison of Pulse Inversion Contrast Harmonic Imaging and Xenon-CT in Evaluation of Brain*
42 *Perfusion*
S. Meairs, P. Horn, R. Kern, J. Beyer, P. Schmiedek, M. Hennerici (Germany)

09.30 *Assessment of Cerebral Perfusion Reserve with Second Harmonic Imaging*
43 J. Federlein, E. Karagiannis, S. Meves, Th. Büttner, H. Przuntek, Th. Postert (Germany)

09.40 *Comparative Visualization of Brain Tissue Perfusion in Various Neurological Disorders Utilizing*
44 *Contrast-Enhanced Harmonic Imaging in Integrated Backscatter and Power Doppler Methods*
T. Shiogai, C. Tsunezuka, M. Koshimura, N. Takayasu, Y. Nagakane, T. Nakase, M. Makino, K. Nakajima, H. Furuhata (Japan)

09.50 *Continuous Measurement of Contrast Induced Signal Enhancement in Transcranial Doppler Examination*
45 *– A Novel Method of Quantitative R/L-Shuntvolume Assessment*
JJ.Schwarze, D.Sander, J.Klingelhöfer (Germany)

10.00 *Indication and Diagnostic Benefit of the Ultrasound Contrast Agent Levovist^R in the Transcranial*
46 *Ultrasound*
P. Zunker, H. Wilms, G. Wasner, A. Allardt, J. A. Zeller. J. Neumann, G. Deuschl (Germany)

10.10 *Benefit of the Ultrasound Contrast Enhancing Agent LevovistR in Patients with Insufficient Temporal*
47 *Bone Window Investigated by Transcranial Doppler Ultrasound*
T. Hansberg, K. S L.Wong, M. A.Ritter, D. W. Droste, E. B. Ringelstein. R. Kay (Hong Kong, Germany)

10.20 *Improved Imaging Quality of Intracranial Vertebrobasilar Arteries by Contrast-Enhanced Colour Duplex*
48 B. Iglseder, W. Staffen, M. Huemer, G. Ladurner (Austria)

Session VIII: 11.00 – 13.00

WORK IN PROGRESS AND FUTURE ASPECTS OF NEUROSONOLOGY

Chairmen: H. FURUHATA, R.G. ACKERSTAFF

Invited Speakers:

11.00 M. HENNERICI
Aspects of Perfusion Measurement in an Acute Stroke Model

11.20 R. AASLID
Recent Progress in Cerebral Hemodynamics

11.40 *Acceleration of Thrombolysis in Vivo by Transcranial Ultrasonication*
49 T. Ishibashi, M. Akiyama, H. Onoue, T. Abe, H. Furuhata (Japan)

11.50 *Non-Invasive Monitoring of Intracranial Pressure and Compliance*
50 K.Paulat, R.Brucher, D.Russell (Norway)

12.00 *Contrast Agent Specific Imaging Modes for the Ultrasonic Assessment of Brain Perfusion*
51 Th. Postert, P. Hoppe, J. Federlein, S. Helbeck, H. Ermert, H. Przuntek, Th. Büttner, W. Wilkening (Germany)

12.10 *Sonographic Brain Tumor Imaging Using Stimulated Acoustic Emission*
52 M. Lange, B. Draganski, F. Schlachetzki, T. Hölscher, L. Kouznetsova, U. Bogdahn (Germany)

12.20 *Volume Flow Changes in the Vertebral Veins during Bilateral Internal Jugular Vein and Circular Neck Compression*
53 J. M. Valdueza, F. Lürtzing, S. J. Schreiber, K. M. Einhäupl (Germany)

12.30 *Reproducibility of Three-Dimensional (3-D) Ultrasound Regarding the Depiction of Carotid Artery Plaque Ulceration*
54 U. Schminke, L.Motsch, C.Kessler (Germany)

12.40 *Detection of the Anterior and Posterior Communicating Artery Using 3D-Transcranial Color-Coded*
55 *Duplexsonography*
Ch. Klötzsch, R. Caspary, G. Lammers, M. Mull, J. Noth (Germany)

12.50 *Patent Foramen Ovale and Internal Jugular Valve Incompetence in Transient Global Amnesia: A Contrast*
56 *Transcranial Doppler Sonography and Color Flow Imaging of Internal Jugular Vein*
A. N. Maalikjy, C. Agosti, G. P. Anzola, E. Morandi, LA.Vignolo, P. Zavrise, A. Padovani (Italy)

SESSION IX : 14.00–16.00

NEUROSONOLOGY AND NEUROIMAGING IN ACUTE STROKE

Chairpersons: E.M. ZANETTE, M. STURZENEGGER

Invited Speakers:

14.00 F. FAZEKAS
MR Techniques in Acute Stroke

14.20 G.M. VON REUTERN
The Neurosonology in Acute Ischemic Stroke (NAIS) Project. Study Design and First Results

14.40 *Hyperdense Middle Cerebral Artery Sign in Occlusion of Middle Cerebral Artery – A Negative Predictor*
57 *for Spontaneous Recanalisation?*
J. Allendoerfer, D. Degner, S. Merx, GM von Reutern (Germany)

14.50 *Prognostic Value of Transcranial Doppler in the Acute Phase of Ischemic Stroke*
58 C. Baracchini, R. Manara, G. Malferrari, B. Marini, M. Del Sette, G. A. Ottonello, G. P. Anzola, L. Lusiani, G. C. Landini, G. Meneghetti (Italy)

15.00 *Sonographic Features of Craniocervical Artery Dissection*
59 A. Lovrencic-Huzjan, M. Bosnar-Puretic, V. Vukovic, V. Demarin (Croatia)

15.10 *Sonographic Monitoring of Midline-Shift in Stroke Patients*
60 E. Stolz, T. Gerriets, I. Fiss, SS. Babacan, C. Algermissen, M. Kaps (Germany)

15.20 *Pattern of Intra- and Extra-Cranial Stenosis in Thai Patients with Stroke and Stroke Risk Factors*
61 D. Ratanakorn, Ch. Dejthevaporn (Thailand)

15.30 *Longitudinal Follow-Up of Intracranial Arterial Stenosis with Transcranial Doppler Ultrasonography*
62 S. U. Kown, J. H. Lee, J. S. Kim (Korea)

15.40 *Thrombolytic Effects of 1 MHZ Standard Diagnostic Ultrasound*
63 K. Spengos, S. Behrens, M. Daffertshofer, C. E. Dempfle, M. Hennerici (Germany)

15.50 *Enhancement of In-Vitro-Thrombolysis by Low-Frequency Ultrasound*
64 M. Nedelmann, B. M Eicke, A. Heimann, O. Kempski, E. Liercke, H. C. Hopf (Germany)

16.00 **Adjourn**

POSTER-SESSION (SESSION V)

Monday, May 22, 2000 14.00–16.00

Hall: Ausstellungshalle and K 1-2

Posters can be mounted on Monday, May 22, starting at 08.00 a.m. and must be taken down on Tuesday, May 23, in the afternoon.

Chairpersons: G. ANZOLA, D. GIOBBE, A. HETZEL, V. OLIVEIRA, P. TRAUBNER, B. ZVAN

See Abstracts 65–171

Cerebrovasc Dis 2000;10(suppl 1):1-44

Abstracts of Oral Presentations

1

AUTOMATED EMBOLI IDENTIFICATION: DETECTION USING A COMBINATION OF TIME AND FREQUENCY DOMAIN INFORMATION

L. Fan, D.H.Evans and A.R. Naylor
Departments of Medical Physics & Surgery, University of Leicester, UK

Emboli can be generally regarded as narrow-band signals with variable bandwidths and central frequencies. They also, in general, have time domain waveforms different from other narrow-band signals such as artifacts and interference. An automated embolus detection system has been designed and implemented off-line, to detect embolic signals using their time and frequency signatures.

FFT based time-frequency analysis is used to pre-select frames containing narrow-band signals as candidate embolic signals. The time domain envelope of each candidate signal is extracted, and six indices which characterise its behavior evaluated. The final signal classification is based on a combination of indices describing the signal bandwidth and central frequency, the energy contained in the narrow band, the energy carried by high frequency components, and the time domain waveform envelope.

The detection system has been tested on a selection of recordings from 21 patients undergoing carotid artery surgery (per-op and post-op) and 4 healthy volunteers. Each of the 32 recordings (seven subjects contributed two recordings each) lasted between 2.5 and 3 minutes giving a total recorded sample length of 85 minutes. The recordings from the patients contained a total of 80 embolic signals (as determined by a human expert) together with 62 intentionally produced artifacts and several periods of diathermy. Using the human expert as a "gold-standard", the automated system demonstrated a sensitivity of 90% and a specificity (for artifact rejection) of approximately 98%. Nine false positive detections occurred during the 85 minutes of recorded signals.

2

A NEW METHOD FOR AUTOMATIC DIFFERENTIATION BETWEEN CEREBRAL EMBOLI AND ARTEFACTS

Rainer Brucher, David Russell. Ulm University of Applied Sciences, Germany and The Dept of Neurology, the National Hospital, Oslo, Norway

Introduction: Cerebral embolus monitoring systems suitable for routine clinical use must have the ability to automatically recognise and differentiate between artefacts and emboli. This has to date proven to be an extremely difficult problem to solve.
Methods: In this study we present a new advancement with regard to the automatic recognition of cerebral emboli and differentiation from artefacts based on a binary decision tree which includes a completely new parameter (BRQ). The latter is the ¼ Doppler shift for the maximum power reflection of an embolic event at 2.5 MHz insonation frequency compared to 2.0 MHz. EmboDop with BRQ software was used in this study of 2000 artefacts and 100 embolic events in one heart valve patient. The level for event recognition was set at 5db above background Doppler power. The artefacts in 2 healthy controls consisted of 200: tapping the probe, 200: tapping the skull, 200: talking (counting), 200: swallowing, 400: coughing, 200: wrinkling the forehead, 200: clenching the teeth, 400: movement of the skin near the probe.
Results: Only two (skin movements near the probe) of the 2000 artefacts were recognised as embolic events. All 100 heart valve emboli were detected and 98 (98%) were correctly classified (specificity 98%).
Conclusion: This study suggests that a binary decision tree including ¼ Doppler shift assessment at 2.0 and 2.5 MHz insonation frequencies will greatly improve the ability to carry out automatic differentiation between artefacts and cerebral emboli during monitoring in routine clinical situations.

3

COMPARISON OF A NEW ON-LINE AUTOMATED EMBOLIC SIGNAL DETECTION ALGORITHM WITH A PANEL OF HUMAN EXPERTS.

M Cullinane, G Reid, R Ackerstaff, V Babikian, D Droste, M Siebler, L Valton, DG Grosset, HS Markus.

St. George's Hospital Medical School, London, UK.

Introduction: The current 'gold standard' for embolic signal (ES) detection is the human expert. Evaluation of a new on-line automated ES detection system was performed by comparing the results from a panel of international human experts against the performance of the software.
Methods: A 2-hour data set from the ipsilateral MCA of 5 patients post-CEA was produced. Identical copies were made and analysed by six independent human experts and the software. The same model of TCD machine was used in each centre and each centre was asked to analyse the recording to their centre standards without the use of an intensity threshold. The time of each ES was recorded and returned to the co-ordinating centre to be analysed. Agreement between centres and the software was performed using the proportion of specific agreement.
Results: A total of 127 ES were recorded by at least one centre. The mean probability of agreement for the six human experts was 0.84. The mean probability of agreement for the six human experts including the software was 0.83.
Conclusion: The performance of the software was equal to that of some individual human experts and only slightly below the mean performance of a panel of human experts.

KARGER
Fax + 41 61 306 12 34
E-Mail karger@karger.ch
www.karger.com
© 2000 S. Karger AG, Basel

4

EVALUATION OF A NEW ON-LINE AUTOMATED EMBOLIC SIGNAL DETECTION ALGORITHM.

R Dittrich, M Cullinane, G Reid, Z Kaposzta, H S Markus.

St. George's Hospital Medical School, London, UK.

Introduction: The clinical applications of TCD for the detection of embolic signals (ES) is limited by the lack of a reliable automated detection system. This study evaluated a new on-line algorithm which utilises the effect of frequency filtering to increase the embolus to blood intensity ratio. It is important to evaluate any new software on all data sets which it will be used. We evaluated it here in patients with carotid stenosis and post-endarterectomy.
Methods: Two data sets were used: 20 hours of data from 21 patients with carotid stenosis and 18 hours of data from 9 patients post carotid endarterectomy (CEA). Each data set was analysed by a human observer and then by the software. All ES detected by the software were matched to the times of the ES detected by the human observer. A decibel threshold of ≥7dB was applied to all data. ES appeared to be more intense in the CEA group.
Results: For the carotid stenosis data 140 ES were detected by the human. At a 65% confidence threshold the software detected 120 true ES and 15 false ES; sensitivity 85.7% and specificity 88.9%. For the post-CEA data 411 ES were detected by the human. At a 65% confidence threshold the software detected 392 true ES and 10 false ES; sensitivity 95.4% and specificity 97.5%.
Conclusion: This automated embolic signal detection system has demonstrated a high level of sensitivity and specificity in two data sets.

5

The Matching Pursuit has the potential to characterize the nature - gaseous or solid - of Microembolic Signals by Transcranial Doppler Ultrasound. ***The Wavelet Study Group.***
G. Devuyst, J-M Vesin, G. de Freitas, N. Cals, N.Afsar, J. Rohr-le-Floch, R. Sztatjzel, J. Serena, C. Molina, M. Ossemann, M. Ritter, D. Droste, EB. Ringelstein, P-A Despland, J. Bogousslavsky.

Background: the aim of this study was to test a new signal processing method called Matching Pursuit (MP) which is related to wavelet transform to characterize the nature - gaseous or solid - of microembolic signals from transcranial Doppler monitoring. The MP provides a very compact representation of the time-frequencies properties of transitory and variable signals such microembolic signals recorded through brain arteries.
Methods: 450 microembolic signals (MES) including 150 presumed solid MES from symptomatic severe internal carotid artery stenosis (>70%), 150 gaseous MES from patients with a patent foramen ovale, and 105 artifacts produce in normal subjects were analyzed in this study. The presumed solid MES came from six different centers (Belgium, Germany, Spain, and Switzerland). For each MES we extracted the time-frequency pattern by an off-line new signal processing tool called Matching Pursuit of the raw data.
Results: Using MP to study the first 75 MES (25 solid, 25 gaseous and 25 artifacts) we have obtained a perfect separation between artifacts and real circulating emboli by the „principal" frequency while two parameters investigating the regularity of the time-frequency representation of MES allowed a perfect distinction of solid MES from gaseous MES. The final analysis is ongoing and complete results will be available at the time of the presentation.
Conclusion: This study has shown that additional signal processing tool such as the Matching Pursuit offers new perspectives to distinguish artifacts from true emboli and to characterize the nature, gaseous or solid, of brain emboli.

6

In vitro evaluation of the mechanism for "tail signs" associated with microembolic signals

E. Furui, K. Hanzawa[1], T. Nakajima[2], N. Fukuhara[2], K. Komai, and M. Yamada

Department of Neurology, Kanazawa University, Kanazawa, Japan
[1]Department of Cardiovascular Surgery, Niigata University, Niigata, Japan
[2]Department of Neurology, National Saigata Hospital, Oogata, Japan

Background and Purpose: We have discovered "tail signs" (TS), a postembolic signal associated with MES which appears as a small reversal signal after MES on the high time resolution spectral display, are specific for MES and can be used as an additional criterion for MES identification. We attempted to determine the mechanism for TS in a flow model and to develop a new diagnostic criterion for MES identification.
Methods: In in vitro flow phantoms with and without an elbow-shaped bend in the downstream segment, we tried to detect MES and TS during injection of microbubbles. After performing TCD monitoring, we did an off-line analysis to investigate the frequency of TS associated with a total of 100 MES. We also examined TS from provoked artifacts.
Results: In the flow phantom with a bend in the downstream segment, all MES were followed by TS. We could find neither TS associated with MES from the flow phantom without a bend, nor TS following artifacts.
Conclusions: TS represent emboli passing down a downstream segment away from the probe. TS are specific for MES and one of the definite criterion for MES identification.

7

MICROEMBOLUS TRACKING WITH POWER M-MODE TRANSCRANIAL DOPPLER ULTRASOUND AND SIMULTANEOUS SINGLE GATE SPECTROGRAM
MA Moehring
BACKGROUND AND PURPOSE: After a decade since the discovery of microembolic signatures in brain blood flow using single gate Doppler ultrasound, microemboli resulting from a variety of pathologies and surgical interventions have been identified. However, the goal of automatic detection of microemboli with high sensitivity and specificity has not been realized with broad acceptance. This work summarizes initial experience with power m-mode Doppler in constructing a platform aimed at more successful automatic detection of microemboli.
METHODS: A 2MHz power m-mode Doppler (Spencer Technologies TCD100M) having 33 sample gates placed at 2 mm intervals from 28 to 92mm depth was configured to display Doppler signal power, colored red and blue for directionality, in an m-mode format. PRF was set to 8kHz and sample volume size was 6mm. Stationary and clutter echoes were assigned no color by rejecting autocorrelation velocities less than 200Hz. The spectrogram for a selected gate depth was displayed simultaneously. 100 embolic signals were collected from a 39 year old male subject with two St. Jude mechanical valves (aortic and mitral). Emphasis was placed on aiming the probe so that the middle cerebral artery and anterior cerebral artery flow signals were visible simultaneously on the m-mode display.
RESULTS: Embolus "tracks" in the m-mode display showed embolic spatial position versus time while the spectrogram showed velocity versus time at the specified gate depth. If and when the embolus track in the m-mode display ran across the spectrogram sample volume depth, the embolus appeared on the spectrogram. In particular, embolic tracks were red and sloped up (motion towards the probe) or blue and sloped down (motion away from the probe). While microemboli showed up distinctly on the m-mode display, clutter artifacts did not.
CONCLUSIONS: These results indicate that automatic detection of microemboli and discrimination from artifacts will be accomplishable on this platform with greater acceptance by the medical community. This work supported by NIH grant 2R44HL57108-02.

8

POSTEMBOLIC SPECTRAL PATTERNS OF MICROEMBOLIC SIGNALS

F Uhlmann*, WJ Schulte-Mattler, D Georgiadis
Departments of Neurology, Martin-Luther University of Halle and Bergmannstrost Klinik (*), Halle / Saale, Germany

Background and Purpose: Postembolic spectral patterns of Doppler microembolic signals (tail- [TS] and lambda-signs [LS]) were described in clinical studies and experimental models. We examined the prevalence of such patterns in MES detected in patients with prosthetic heart valves. Patients and Methods: Ten patients with prosthetic heart valves (7 men and 3 women, age 57±8 years, mitral valve replacement, n=2, aortic valve replacement, n=5, dual valve replacement, n=3) were bilaterally monitored with transcranial Doppler ultrasound, using a pulsed ultrasound machine (Multi-Dop X-4, DWL, Sipplingen) over both middle cerebral arteries and data saved on DAT tapes for later reevaluation. Additionally, artifact signals were produced during TCD monitoring of 5 normal controls by speaking, chewing, swallowing or tapping of the transducer. MES and artifacts were identified by two independent observers and also by the TCD 8 software (version 8T). Only signals unanimously identified by the human observers and the software were further evaluated. Tail sign was defined as unequivocal reverse signals, appearing on the high time resolution spectral display within 75 mseconds after the MES, while lamda sign was defined as a Doppler frequency shift resembling the letter lambda and appearing on the high time resolution spectral display within 25 mseconds after the MES. Results: A total of 1721 MES and 733 artifact signals were identified. TS and LS were observed after 168 MES (9.8%) and 190 MES (11%), respectively. No TS or LS were observed after any of the 733 artifact signals. Conclusions: LS and TS are highly specific for MES. Their low prevalence though, substantially reduces their potential use as an additional differentiation criterion between MES and artifact signals.

9

ASYMPTOMATIC CAROTID EMBOLI STUDY (ACES)

Hugh Markus and Marisa Cullinane for the ACES Investigators
Division of Clinical Neuroscience, St.George's Hospital Medical School, Cranmer Terrace, London, SW17 0RE, UK
Email: h.markus@sghms.ac.uk

Background

Operating on an unselected group of patients with asymptomatic carotid stenosis, offers poor risk benefit ratios. Techniques are required to select a high risk group who may particularly benefit from operation. Pilot studies suggest that the presence of asymptomatic cerebral emboli detected by Doppler Ultrasound may identify a high risk group.

Method

The Asymptomatic Carotid Emboli Study is an international multi-centre study of 600 patients with asymptomatic carotid stenosis. Transcranial Doppler ultrasound recordings are made for 1 hour from the ipsilateral middle cerebral artery on two occasions at study entry. Recordings on DAT tape are forwarded to the co-ordinating centre for central analysis which allows blinding to the results of embolic signal monitoring. Patients are followed at 6 monthly intervals for 2 years. Where possible recordings are repeated at 6 months, 12 months, and 18 months. There is an optional arm which includes performing reactivity measurements at study onset. The primary outcome measure is ipsilateral stroke in the territory of the stenosis carotid artery.

The study is funded by the British Heart Foundation and has recently started. The collaborators are keen to enrol further centres. It is expected to finish in 2003.

10

ASYMPTOMATIC STENOSIS EMBOLUS DETECTION (ASED) STUDY

A Harris, B Chambers, J Stork, C Levi, C Bladin, G Donnan.
Neurology Department, Austin & Repatriation Medical Centre, Heidelberg West, Victoria, Australia, 3081
Presenter; A Harris

Meta analysis of carotid endarterect-omy (CEA) trials in asymptomatic patients shows at best a weak surgical benefit. Identification of high-risk patients would increase the benefit. TCD detection of microemboli is a valid technique for predicting stroke or TIA after carotid endarterectomy and so is potentially useful for patients with asymptomatic carotid stenosis. The aim of ASED is to test the hypothesis that transcranial Doppler (TCD) detection of microemboli distal to asymptomatic internal carotid artery (ICA) stenosis can identify patients at higher risk of ipsilateral stroke.

Patients with asymptomatic 60-99% ICA stenosis by carotid duplex (CD) criteria and no other apparent source of cerebral emboli undergo six monthly CD, 60minute ipsilateral middle cerebral artery TCD recording and clinical assessment. Off-line six decibel threshold microemboli counts are correlated with the primary out-come of ipsilateral carotid transient ischaemic attack, stroke or stroke-death. The estimated sample size is 500 arteries. 160 patients with 180 eligible arteries (35% with 80-99% stenosis) have attended up to seven visits each. Thirty-four (19%) different arteries have been microemboli positive on at least one occasion with counts up to seven per hour. 70 arteries have been monitored at least thrice; 49 were consistently emboli-negative, 16 were positive once, 5 were positive twice and none positive more than twice. Seven patients have had primary outcome events and three of these were emboli positive prior.

Preliminary data support the hypothesis that TCD detection of microemboli distal to asymptomatic carotid artery stenosis can identify patients at higher risk of ipsilateral TIA or stroke.

11

CEREBRAL MICROEMBOLISM CORRESPONDS TO ANTIPLATELET MEDICATION IN PATIENTS WITH SYMPTOMATIC ARTERIAL STENOSIS

S. Krueger, T. Blaser, C.-W. Wallesch, M. Goertler
Department of Neurology
Otto-von-Guericke University Magdeburg, Germany

Background: Microemboli detected by transcranial Doppler in patients with symptomatic arterial stenosis are associated with an increased risk of recurrent stroke. Antithrombotic agents, of proven efficacy in stroke prevention mainly through reduction of cerebral embolism, have not shown an impact on microemboli yet.
Patients and Methods: From 192 consecutively referred patients with symptomatic arterial stenosis in the anterior circulation and clinical symptoms within the last 30 days, 74 (50 men; mean age 60.1+/-14 years) underwent one-hour bilateral embolus detection. Patients were excluded if they had insufficient bone windows (n=42) or if embolus detection could not be organised without an antithrombotic medication excepting acetylsalicylic acid (n=76). With exception of higher age and a higher frequency of women in patients with an insufficient bone window, selected and excluded patients did not differ by their clinical characteristics.
Results. The absence of an antiplatelet prevention at the time of the embolus detection (OR 7.1, 95%CI 1.6-31.4, p=0.010), an extracranial localisation of the stenosis (OR 7.1, 95%CI 1.6-32.7, p=0.011) and recurrent ischemic events (OR 3.8, 95%CI 1.1-13.3, p=0.038) were independent predictors for microemboli. Patients with and without microemboli did not differ by their age, sex, risk factors, type of symptoms, CT/MRT findings, degree of stenosis and time between ischemia and embolus detection.
Conclusions: Detection of microemboli in patients with recently symptomatic arterial stenosis is associated with the absence of an antiplatelet medication, suggesting an influence of antiplatelet drugs on microemboli of presumed arterial origin.

12

DOPPLER MICROEMBOLIC SIGNALS DURING CARDIAC SURGERY

D Georgiadis, R Stets, A Schorcht, A Hempel, F Uhlmann, G Fischer, RE Silber (*), HR Zerkowski (*), S Zierz
Departments of Neurology and of Cardiothoracic Surgery (*), Martin-Luther University of Halle, Halle / Saale, Germany

Background and Purpose: We evaluated incidence and counts of MES during cardiac surgery, and their relation to clinical and operative parameters. Patients and Methods: TCD monitoring was performed in 97 patients (77 men, 20 women, age 60±10 years) undergoing cardiac surgery for valve replacement (n=12), coronary artery bypass (CABG, n=78) or both (n=7) over both MCAs. The operative procedure was subdivided in 4 phases (I-skin incision to cannulation of the aorta, II-cannulation of the aorta until begin of cardiopulmonary bypass [CPB], III- CPB, IV- opening of the aortic clamp till end of reperfusion period). Five patients were retrospectively excluded from further evaluation. Serum levels of S-100ß and neuron specific enolase (NSE) were evaluated in 25 patients preoperatively, as well as in the first 5 postoperative days. Additionally, 10 patients were monitored over both MCAs and before and behind the arterial filter of the membrane oxygenator. All data was saved on digital audio tapes. Results: Significant differences in MES prevalence and counts were noted among the different monitoring periods, and between patients undergoing CABG and those undergoing surgery for valve replacement (353 [260-515] versus 3147 [866-5015] respectively, p<0.0001). Significantly higher MES counts / CPB minute were noted when a DIDECO oxygenator (DIDECO SA, Mirandola, Italy) was used, as compared to use of a COBE (Cobe Lab., Lakewood, CO) oxygenator (5.7 [2.6-8.4], n=37 versus 0.9 [0.5-1.3], n=55, respectively, p<0.0001). A trend towards higher total MES counts was observed in patients with postoperative neurological deficit (n=9) as compared to remaining cases (972 [146-5901] versus 572 [400-884], respectively, p=0.7). No relation between NSE or S-100ß levels and MES counts was noted. A dramatic reduction in MES was noted when comparing counts detected before the oxygenator filter to those detected behind the filter and in the MCAs (7917 [4927-15844], 4643 [2916-10411] and 282 [47-1108] respectively). Conclusions: MES counts during cardiac surgery depend on the type of operation and oxygenator, and are not related to postoperative S-100ß or NSE levels. Only approximately 4% of emboli produced by the oxygenator finally reach the brain.

13

ANTIPLATELETS REDUCED NON-GASEOUS HITS IN PATIENTS WITH MECHANICAL VALVE

Kazuhiko Hanzawa, Eisuke Furui*, Satoshi Namura, Hisanaga Moro, Masaya Kitamura, Takashi Nakajima**, Nobuyoshi Fukuhara**, Jun-ichi Hayashi, Hiroaki Naritomi***
Cardiothrac. Surg. Niigata University School of Medicine,* Neurology, Kanazawa University School of Medicine, Neurology, **National Saigata Hospital, ***National Cardiovascular Center, JAPAN

Purpose: The significance of HITS in patients with mechanical valve is still controversial. We attempted to elucidate whether antiplatelets reduce non-gaseous HITS determined by oxygen inhalation methods.

Methods: Forty four patients with mechanical valve replacement were subjected. All the patients had only anticoagulation therapy. HITS were detected by TC2020 with 2.0 MHz for 15 min before oxygen inhalation. The oxygen was inhaled through a face mask for 10 min, and thereafter HITS were detected under oxygen inhalation for the following 15 min. Patients without HITS reduction by oxygen inhalation underwent antiplatelet therapy (200 mg ticlopidine) for a month and were examined again in the same way after the therapy.

Results: In a group as a whole, HITS count was significantly reduced by oxygen inhalation (18±16/15 min to 7±12/15 min) (p<0.0001). However, HITS count was unchanged in 6 patients with TIA or thrombus formation in the heart. In these patients , HITS decreased significantly from 14±9/15 min to 4±4/15 min following the antiplatelet therapy (p<0.05).

Comments: Most HITS in mechanical valve patients may reflect cavitation bubbles. Oxygen inhalation methods can distinguish micro-thrombus and bubble s. This method may be useful for decision making of additional antiplatelet therapy in order to prevent cerebral embolism after mechanical valve replacement.

14

PATENT FORAMEN OVALE AND OBSTRUCTIVE APNEA SYNDROME

M. Del Sette, S. Angeli, F. Ferrillo[1], M. Beelke[1], L. Nobili[1], S. Pretta, C. Gandolfo.
Department of Neurosciences and Vision and [1]Center of Sleep Medicine, DISMR, University of Genova, Italy.

High prevalence (69%) of patent foramen ovale (PFO) has been recently described in subjects with obstructive apnea syndrome (OSA). The aim of our study was to evaluate the prevalence of PFO diagnosed by transcranial Doppler in OSA at rest, during Valsalva manouvre and during sleep.

We evaluted 50 subjects with OSA (35 males, 5 females) and compared them with 76 control subjects without history of migraine (36 males and 40 females). All the subjects underwent transcranial doppler (Multidop DWL, Sipplingen, Germany) with injection of contrast medium in an antecubital vein (agitated solution of 9 ml saline and 1 ml of air). The test was performed with patients at rest and during Valsalva manouvre. In subjects with large PFO (more than 20 bubbles) a polysomnographic registration was performed with transcranial Doppler testing for FO patency during sleep.

Thirteen out of the 50 OSA had PFO (26%), as opposed to twelve of the 76 controls (16%) (p=0.2); in both groups PFO was present mainly during Valsalva (11/13 OSA, 83% and 10/12 controls, 80%). In the 4 subjects with large shunt the test performed during sleeping apnea showed presence of shunt during apnoea, with a smaller amount of bubbles compared to Valsalva manouvre.

Prevalence of PFO in subjects with OSA is not-significantly higher than in normal controls, and the shunt is frequently present only during Valsalva (83%). In the nocturnal sleeping period, subjects with large shunts show passage of bubbles through the foramen ovale.

15

GPIIb/IIIa Platelet Receptor Antagonists in Acute Ischemic Stroke

Mario Siebler, Ulrich Junghans, und Seitz R.
Department of Neurology, Heinrich-Heine-University Düsseldorf

Platelet activation and aggregation play a major role in arterial thrombus formation which is the leading cause of cerebral ischemia. Large double-blind, placebo controlled clinical trials have well documented that platelet GPIIb/IIIa receptor antagonists are effective drugs in unstable angina and non-Q-wave myocardial infarction. In acute stroke, only thrombolysis with intravenously administered recombinant tissue plasminogen activator (rtPA) has been shown to improve clinical outcome but this therapy has clear limitations concerning the risk of intracerebral bleeding and the narrow therapeutic time- window within a few hours after symptom onset.

We investigated 15 consecutive stroke patients (11 men, median age 56 years) who were admitted within 3 to 12 hours after symptom onset to our Stroke Unit and deteriorated progressively. Diffusion weighted magnetic resonance imaging depicted acute small or moderate ischemic lesions in the territory of the middle cerebral (MCA, n=9), posterior cerebral (PCA, n=1) and vertebro-basilar artery (BA,n=4) compatible with the recent neurological deficits. While under intravenous heparin (1000 IE/hr) they all continued to show progressive or fluctuating neurological symptoms. In two patients angiography revealed an occlusion of the basilar artery. Although, these 2 patients were immediately treated with rtPA (20mg /50 mg, respectively), they clinically deteriorated further.

Tirofiban was given intravenously using 0,4 µg/kg/min loading dose for 30 minutes followed by a 0,1 µg/kg/min infusion with heparin for at least 24 hours in all 15 patients. Microembolidetection using transcranial Doppler sonography could be performed in 11 subjects before study treatment and 5 of them displayed microembolic signals. Corresponding to the pharmacodynamic the event rates dropped significantly to zero within 30 minutes and remained low during the infusion time. All but one patients displayed clinical stabilisation or even improvement within the next days. The 2 patients with basilar occlusion improved dramatically after application of tirofiban within 30-60 minutes. Control CT scans excluded intracranial haemorrhage in all patients.

The effect of tirofiban on the ME rate supports the concept that ME are composed by formed elements. We conclude, that GPIIb/IIIa antagonists may have a substantial potential in acute stroke therapy either to support thrombolysis or to bridge the time of „unstable" cerebral ischemia, a concept similar to that proven effective in coronary artery disease.

16

S-NITROSOGLUTATHIONE, A PLATELET SPECIFIC NITRIC OXIDE DONOR, AND L-ARGININE REDUCE EMBOLISATION POST CAROTID ENDARTERECTOMY

Z Kaposzta, PA Baskerville, SCA Fraser, D Madge, JF Martin, HS Markus. Clinical Neuroscience, St. George's Hospital Medical School (ZK, HSM); Vascular Surgery King's College Hospital (PAB, SCAF); University College of London (DM, JFM), London, UK

Introduction: Asymptomatic cerebral embolic signals (ES) are common after carotid endarterectomy (CEA). A high frequency of ES during the early postoperative phase predicts early stroke and TIA risk. S-Nitrosoglutathione (GSNO), a nitric oxide (NO) donor which may have relative platelet specificity. GSNO administered during CEA, starting from the induction of anaesthesia until 2 hours after skin closure reduced the rate of embolisation. However it caused some intraoperative hypotensive episodes. L-Arginine (L-Arg) is a NO precursor, which may inhibit platelet aggregation by the formation of cyclic GMP. The aims of this study were to determine whether 1) GSNO reduced embolisation when administered postoperatively only and, 2) post-operative L-Arg also reduced embolisation.

Methods and results: Transcranial Doppler ultrasound (TCD) recordings from the ipsilateral middle cerebral artery were made in patients randomised double-blind to placebo (N=13), GSNO (N=10), or L-Arg (N=13) given IV from 30 min to 2 hours after skin closure. Data was recorded onto DAT for blinded analysis. Both GSNO and L-Arg reduced embolisation for up to 24 hours. GSNO almost abolished ES.

	Median (range) of embolic signals (ES/h)		
	postop 0-4 hrs	6-7 hrs	24-25 hrs
GSNO	*0.8(0-8)	‡0(0)	§0(0)
L-Arg	†9.9(0-225)	‡1.5(0-5)	0(0-1)
Placebo	47.8(6-778)	22.6(0-188)	5.3(0-38)

*P<0.0001; †P=0.002; ‡P=0.01; §P=0.03 versus placebo

Conclusions: GSNO is effective when administered postoperatively, and the hypotensive episodes seen with intraoperative administration were not seen in this study. L-Arg also reduced the rate of embolisation. This indicates that L-Arg has a clinically significant antiplatelet effect in man. Our results suggest the potential use of these drugs in the treatment of thromboembolic disease.

17

CAN INTIMA-MEDIA TICKNESS PREDICT RISK OF STROKE IN PATIENTS WITH ACUTE MYOCARDIAL INFARCTION ?

V Oliveira, A Pedro, P Batista, F Soares.
Dept. Neurology, Hospital S. Maria, Lisboa, Portugal.

Introduction: Intima-media tickness (IMT) is a non-invasive ultrasonographic method that has been used to assess atherosclerosis. Several studies have found a positive association between increase in IMT and some vascular risk factors, although those associations are not uniformly found. Since myocardial infarction (MI) and Ischemic non-embolic stroke are consequences of atherosclerosis, we looked for IMT in those patients.

Patients and Methods: One hundred and fifty patients with diagnosis of acute myocardial infarction admitted to a coronary unit were studied. Color Duplex sonography was obtained as part of the routine work-up to assess carotid bifurcations. Measurements of IMT were also obtained bilaterally from the far wall of the distal segments of internal carotid arteries, within 0,8 mm as described elsewhere. Several measurements were obtained in each side and then the average was made.

Results: A positive association between increase in IMT and the following variables were seen: age, male gender, diabetes and smoking.

In patients with in-hospital or past history of cerebrovascular ischemic events (6.7%), an association was also found with IMT, been more significant for recent in hospital events (4 %) than for past history (2.7%).

Conclusion: In our population IMT is influenced by some known vascular risk factors (age, male gender, diabetes and smoking). Although limited by the reduced number of the sample, patients with MI who had evidence of ischemic cerebrovascular events presented higher IMT values.

18

REDUCED PROGRESSION OF EARLY ATHEROSCLEROSIS FOLLOWING ANTIBIOTIC THERAPY AFTER ISCHEMIC STROKE AND CHLAMYDIA PNEUMONIAE SEROPOSITIVITY

D. Sander, K. Winbeck, J. Klingelhöfer*, B. Heyse, J. Schwarze*, B. Conrad
Dept. of Neurology, Technical University of Munich and *Klinikum Chemnitz, Germany

Chlamydia pneumoniae (Cp) infection has been associated with atherosclerosis and has been proposed as a possible additional cardiovascular risk factor. Some studies indicate a possible beneficial effect of antibiotic therapy on future cardiovascular events in Cp seropositivity.

We evaluated the effect of roxithromycin therapy according to the ROXXIS study protocol on the progression of the intima to media-thickness (IMT) of the common carotid artery using duplex untrasonography in a prospective study with a follow-up of at least 2 years (mean: 2.4 years) in 292 consecutive patients with ischemic stroke aged over 55 years in whom the first IMT measurement and the Cp testing (IgG and IgA) was performed at least 3 years before the beginning of roxithromycin therapy.

CP IgG antibodies (> 1:128) were initially found in 123 (42%) patients and IgA antibodies (≥ 1:16) in 119 (40.8%) patients. In the 3 years before the onset of antibiotic therapy, patients with serological detection of Cp showed a significant enhanced progression of the IMT even after adjustment for other cardiovascular risk factors (0.12 mm/year [95% confidence interval 0.10; 0.15] vs. 0.06 mm/year [0.03; 0.09]; p<0.001). The 61 CP positive patients given roxithromycin showed a significantly decreased IMT progression after 2 years compared to the Cp positive patients without therapy (0.07 mm/year vs. 0.11 mm/year, p<0.01). However, no significant difference in the occurrence of future cardiovascular events was found between both groups during the follow-up period. No change of IMT was observed in Cp negative patients given roxithromycin (n=84), compared to those without therapy (0.05 vs. 0.06 mm/year).

Our findings suggest a possible positive impact of antibiotic therapy on early atherosclerosis progression in Cp seropositive patients with cerebrovascular disease.

19

ELEVATED C-REACTIVE PROTEIN IS ASSOCIATED WITH AN INCREASED EARLY ATHEROSCLEROSIS.

K. Winbeck, Ch. Kukla, B. Heyse, *J. Klingelhöfer, B. Conrad, D. Sander
Department of Neurology, Technical University Munich and *Klinikum Chemnitz, Germany

Elevated C reactive protein (CRP) is known to be an independent risk factor for the development of cardiovascular diseases. In this study we analyzed the relationship between serum CRP levels and early atherosclerosis.

We evaluated the intima to media wall thickness (IMT) of the common carotid artery in 315 consecutive neurological in-patients (156 male mean age 64.4 years [95% confidence interval (CI): 63; 66] years) using high-resolution Duplex ultrasonography. 174 patients had a history of a cerebral ischemic event. The baseline CRP concentration was determined within 24 hours after hospitalization. Patients with elevated CRP due to acute or recently treated infections were excluded from analysis. Patients were subdivided according to normal (<0.5 mg/dl) and increased CRP concentration. No significant differences regarding age, pack-years of smoking, cholesterol and triglycerides were found between the two subgroups. Patients with an elevated CRP showed a significant larger IMT (1.07 [1.03; 1.11] vs. 0.93 [0.90; 0.96]). Moreover, significant differences were found for gender, body mass index, HDL cholesterol, incidence of arterial hypertension, carotid plaques and known ischemic stroke. Multivariate linear regression analysis revealed an elevated baseline CRP level as an independent risk factor for an increased IMT (p=0.027).

Elevated CRP is an independent risk factor for early carotid atherosclerosis measured with B mode ultrasonography. Our data support the importance of chronic inflammation for the early stages of atherosclerosis formation.

20

INCREASED CAROTID ARTERY INTIMA-MEDIA THICKNESS IN U.K. AFRICAN CARIBBEANS

Z Kaposzta, M Cullinane, R Dittrich, C Wolfe, HS Markus

St George's and GKT Medical Schools, London, UK

Introduction Stroke incidence is double in UK African Caribbean's (AC) compared with Caucasians. Increased arterial damage in response to cardiovascular risk factors might partially explain this. An estimate of early arterial damage and atherosclerosis can be obtained from common carotid artery (CCA) intima-media thickness (IMT).

Methods and Results 291 males (89 AC, 202 Caucasian) aged 42-77 yr. (mean 61.5) were randomly selected from family practices in South London. An image of CCA posterior wall was captured on duplex ultrasound. Images were digitised and analysed blinded to case identity using a semi-automated computer programme measuring mean IMT over a 1-2 cm segment. Mean (SD) CCA IMT was increased in AC: 0.82(0.16) v 0.75(0.13)mm, p<0.0001. After controlling for cardiovascular risk factors and manual occupation with multiple regression IMT was still increased in AC (regression coefficient 0.043 mm, p=0.022). Increased IMT was also associated with age (p=0.0001), BMI (p=0.007), systolic BP (p=0.0005), diastolic BP (p=0.007), diabetes mellitus (p=0.008). When factors of childhood socio-economic status (absence of hot water, no of rooms in house, inside bathroom, no of people in house) were also entered the strength of the association with AC ethnicity was reduced (coefficient 0.034 mm, p=0.09).

Conclusion CCA IMT is increased in UK AC after controlling for cardiovascular risk factors. The association was reduced when markers of childhood socio-economic deprivation were controlled for. This may be due to confounding by previously uncontrolled adult socio-economic factors, but could reflect childhood socio-economic factors influencing adult arterial disease perhaps by factors such as chronic infection and chronic inflammation.

21

Intima-media thickness and Ambulatory Blood Pressure Monitoring in hypertensive patients.

C. Barone, *F. Nobili, N.R. Musso, V. De Iorgi, F. #Copello, G. Lotti, *G. Rodriguez.

Clinical Medicine III, *Clinical Neurophysiology Serv. (Dept. Internal Medicine) #Dept. of Occupational Medicine (S. Martino Hosp.), Genoa, Italy.

The effect of 24-hour Ambulatory Blood Pressure Monitoring (ABPM) parameters on Intima-Media Thickness (IMT) is currently widely investigated. However, the relationship between IMT and Blood Pressure (BP) values with respect to the day-night cycle is not still fully elucidated. Fifty-seven hypertensive patients (47 treated, 10 untreated; 25 men, 32 women, mean age: 55± 12) underwent continuous ABPM for 24 hours. Nine BP variables were considered: mean systolic, diastolic, and Mean Arterial BP (MABP) values during the day, the night, and over 24 hours, respectively. Within 1 month from ABPM, patients underwent Duplex scanning of neck vessels. IMT was measured at the last centimetre of the Common Carotid Artery (CCA) before the bifurcation. In each side, IMT was measured at three levels in the anterior and lateral CCA, thus obtaining 6 measures in each side. The twelve IMT values were then averaged to obtain a single mean IMT value. Multivariate Analysis of Variance showed IMT to be significantly related (r^2= 0.3) to the three nocturnal BP values only. These data highlight the relevance of nocturnal BP values as compared to diurnal and 24-hour values.

22

AGING DEPENDENT DECREASE IN THE CEREBRAL AUTOREGULATION AFTER ADRENERGIC STIMULATION BY HAND-GRIP

S. Castellani *, I. Carobbi **, N. Boni *,V. Corsoni *,F. Lavorini***,C. Zeloni *, F. Battaglia*, G.F. Gensini *, G. Masotti **

Dipartimento di area critica medica e chirurgica -*Sez. Clinica Medica Generale e Cardiologia; ** Sez. Gerontologia Geriatria e Clinica Urologica; *** Sez Medicina Respiratoria, University of Florence, Italy

A defect in pressure autoregulation has been described in different disease states as essential hypertension. It is not known whether a distinct pattern of pressure autoregulation may also characterize some physiological conditions; in particular it is not known whether aging itself can modify the adaptation of cerebral blood flow to pressor stimuli. The aim of this study was to evaluate the effect of aging on the autoregulation capacity of the cerebral blood flow in response to an adrenergic stimulation with hand-grip, a stimulus known to increase arterial blood pressure. 10 young healthy normotensives (age 21 to 31 yrs, mean 24,5), and 10 healthy elderly subjects (age 60 to 69 yrs, mean 64,5) were studied. They were all non smokers, had a BMI<27, and were not offspring of diabetic or hypertensive patients. Cerebral hemodynamics was bilaterally investigated with transcranial Doppler (MultiDop x 4 DWL) by measuring the mean velocity in the middle cerebral artery (MCA) through the temporal windows by two 2 MHz probes. Arterial blood pressure (Finapres) and CO_2 (Datex Normocap CO_2 monitor) were simultaneously recorded. During the whole experiment all subjects were studied in a supine position. After a 30 minute baseline stabilization period all subjects performed a 90 sec right hand grip stimulation. The hand grip was followed by a recovery period that lasted until all hemodynamic variables had reverted to baseline. Hand grip induced a significant blood pressure increase in both groups (+13% at peak, vs baseline, p<0.04 in the young; +16.8% vs. baseline, p <0.005 in the elderly). CO_2 did not vary in either group. Vm in the MCA did not change. in the young. In the elderly, the stimulus caused on both sides a significant increase in Vm during the whole experimental period until 15 minutes after the stimulus cessation (F= 4.10 ; p<0.0001 for both sides) (p<0.025 vs baseline in left MCAat peak ; p<0,03 vs baseline in the right MCA at peak). Pressure autoregulation was effective in the young but was lacking in the elderly in whom similar increases in arterial blood pressure were associated with an increase in Vm extending beyond the application of the stimulus. Given the excess in blood pressure variability observed in the elderly, this lack of pressure autoregulation can represent a mechanism of vascular damage and facilitate the ischemic events which are observed more often. among the aged.

23

IMPAIRED CEREBROVASCULAR REACTIVITY PREDICTS STROKE AND TIA RISK IN CAROTID ARTERY DISEASE; A PROSPECTIVE STUDY

M Cullinane, HS Markus.

St George's Hospital Medical School, London, UK

Background: Cross sectional studies suggest impaired cerebral haemodynamics is associated with symptomatic status in carotid stenosis and occlusion but there is little prospective data.

Methods: Transcranial Doppler was used to determine middle cerebral artery reactivity to 8% carbon dioxide in air in 107 patients with either carotid occlusion (N=48) or asymptomatic carotid stenosis (N=59). Subjects were prospectively followed for a mean duration of 634 days. No patients dropped out due to operation prior to symptoms or due to loss of contact.

Results: There were 11 ispilateral ischaemic events during follow up (6 stroke, 5 TIA), and 7 non-stroke deaths. Severely reduced ipsilateral MCA reactivity (<20% flow velocity increase), predicted ipsilateral stroke and TIA risk in the whole group (Kaplan-Meier p<0.0001), and in occlusion (p=0.005) and stenosis (p=0.015) groups alone. It also predicted risk of ipsilateral stroke alone in all three groups. Cox regression was performed controlling for age, gender, hypertension, diabetes, current smoking, ipsilateral CT infarct contralateral stenosis%, and ipsilateral stenosis v occlusion. Only impaired reactivity (OR 12.2, 95% CI 2.38-62.92, p=0.002) and female gender (p=0.004) independently predicted ipsilateral stroke and TIA risk.

Conclusions: Severely reduced cerebrovascular reactivity predicts stroke and TIA risk in both carotid stenosis and occlusion.

24

DETECTION OF CIRCLE OF WILLIS COLLATERALS: MRA COMPARED TO TRANSCRANIAL DUPLEX SCANNING

A.W.J. Hoksbergen[1], D.A. Legemate[1], C.B.L.M. Majoie[2], F.J.H. Hulsmans[2]
Depts. of Vascular Surgery[1] and Radiology[2], Academic Medical Center Amsterdam, The Netherlands

Aim: To compare magnetic resonance angiography (MRA) with transcranial color-coded duplex sonography (TCCD) as reference standard for the detection of non-recruited circle of Willis collaterals.
Methods: In 50 healthy volunteers, 25 men and 25 women with a mean age of 50 (28-74) the collateral potential of the anterior (AcoA) and posterior (PcoA) communicating arteries was tested by TCCD and carotid compression. The criteria to define AcoA and PcoA function were respectively, reversal of flow in the A1-segment of the anterior cerebral artery and a peak systolic velocity increase >20% in the P1-segment of the posterior cerebral artery during ipsilateral carotid compression. Next, subjects underwent three-dimensional time-of-flight MRA. Collaterals were defined as functionally patent if they were visible on the MR angiogram. The results were reviewed in a blinded fashion. The sensitivity and specificity of MRA in detecting AcoA and PcoA patency was determined.
Results: TCCD defined 2 (4%) AcoAs and 16 (16%) PcoAs as non-functional. MRA failed to visualize 8 (16%) AcoAs and 23 (23%) PcoAs. The table shows the overall sensitivity and specificity of MRA for the detection of non-recruited but functional communicating arteries (n=150).

Table: MRA versus TCCD

AcoA+PcoA		*TCCD*			
		yes	no		
MRA	yes	115	4	Sensitivity=87%	PPV=97%
	no	17	14	Specificity=78%	NPV=45%

PPV=positive predictive value, NPV=negative predictive value

Conclusion: Compared to TCCD, MRA has a moderate to high level of sensitivity and specificity in detecting patency of non-recruited collateral arteries of the circle of Willis. This raises the question whether MRA is sufficiently adequate to test the functional capacity of the circle of Willis.

25

Intraoperative transcranial Doppler monitoring and the prediction of stroke from carotid endarterectomy.

R.G.A. Ackerstaff[1], M.P. Spencer[4], C.J.W. van de Vlasakker[2], F.L. Moll[1], F.E.E. Vermeulen[1], A. Algra[3], G.M. Moons[3].

From the (1) St. Antonius Hospital, Nieuwegein (Utrecht), (2) Slingeland Hospital, Doetinchem, and (3) Julius Center for General Practice and Patient Oriented Research, University Medical Center Utrecht, The Netherlands, and from (4) Spencer Technologies, Seattle, USA.

Purpose. In a pooled data analysis of 1058 patients who underwent elective carotid endarterectomy (CEA), we evaluated which intraoperative transcranial Doppler (TCD) emboli and velocity variables were independently associated with operative stroke and stroke related death, using a multivariable logistic regression model and Receiver Operating Characteristic (ROC) curve analysis. Moreover, the independent impact of various preoperative patients characteristics on outcome was also assessed.
Results. Thirty-nine (3.7%) of our patients developed a stroke. Four of these patients died. In the final prediction model, emboli during dissection (odds ratio (OR) 1.50; 95% confidence interval (CI) 0.77-2.93) and during wound closure (OR 2.27; 95% CI 1.16-4.43) as well as ≥ 90% decrease of middle cerebral artery (MCA) blood flow velocity at cross-clamping (OR 3.31; 95% CI 1.28-8.54) and ≥ 100% pulsatility index increase at clamp release (OR 7.06; 95% CI 1.39-35.73) were independently associated with operative stroke. Of the patient characteristics, preoperative cerebral ischaemia (OR 1.89; 95% CI 0.97-3.69) and ≥ 70% ipsilateral internal carotid artery stenosis (OR 0.46; 95% CI 0.23-0.93) were also associated with outcome. The ROC area of this model was 0.73.
Conclusion. The combination of TCD detected microembolism during dissection and wound closure with significant MCA velocity changes at cross-clamping and clamp release and the presence of preoperative cerebral symptoms and ≥ 70% ipsilateral internal carotid artery stenosis reasonably discriminates between patients with and without operative stroke. This makes intraoperative TCD monitoring useful to stratify patients during surgery according to their risk of operative stroke and can help the surgeon to improve his or her technique.

26

ARE CAROTID STENTS A SOURCE OF MICROEMBOLI LATE AFTER DEPLOYMENT ?

B. Censori, T. Partziguian, L. Casto, M. Camerlingo, A. Mamoli.
Neurologia 2 - Ospedali Riuniti - Bergamo - ITALY.

Objective. To assess if carotid stents are a source of Doppler microemboli (MES) months to years after deployment. MES may indicate a late embolic risk from the stents. **Patients and Methods.** We have studied two groups of patients at different intervals after deployment of Wallstents or Palmaz stents for ≥ 50% carotid stenosis. Group 1 included 19 patients studied 6 to 12 months after stenting (median 8 months); group 2 included 17 patients studied > 12 months after stenting (median 26 months; range 15 to 39 months). The TCD probe was manually held at the temporal window ipsilateral to the stented artery for 35 to 50 minutes without interruption, focussing on the middle cerebral artery at ad depth of 46 to 54 mm. **Results.** Only 1 of 19 patients in Group 1 showed MES (0.5%), in a large number. However, this patient had mechanical aortic and mitral valves and showed many MES also on recording from the common carotid artery below the stent. Therefore, his MES were probably of cardiac origin. No patient in Group 2 showed any MES. **Conclusions.** Carotid stents do not seem to be a source of microemboli months to years after their deployment. This is a reassuring information for present and future patients harboring such stents.

27

The Risk Factors of Severe Brain Ischania (SBI) during Carotid Endarterectomia (CE) and ICA clamping.

V.A.Shakhnovich, V.A.Lazarev, G.E.Mitroshin, M.V.Churilov, D.Y.Usachev, A.A.Shmigelsky, A.Y.Lubnin
Burdenko Neurosurgery Institute, Moscow, Russia.

Aim: Preoperetive assessment of risk factors which can lead to SBI during CE.
Material and Methods: Perioperative monitoring of FV in both MCA´s was performed in 39 pts with symptomatic carotid stenosis (m 36, age 46-67y) having undergone a total CE due stenosis of ICA of 50-95%. The contralateral ICA was normal in 21 pts, stenosed/occluded in 11/7 pts. Extracranial and transcranial Color Coded Duplex was used to assess the size of carotid plaques and patency of Circle of Willis, the anterior communicating artery (a com AQ) and posterior communicating artery (P com A). The perantage reduction of FV in MCA on TCD during clamping ICA upon CE measured reserve capacity of collateral circulation, caused mainly by the state of Circle of Willis, contralateral ICA and VA. Cerebrovascular reactivity (CVR) was assessed by 1g. Acetazolamide application and evaluation of percentage changes of FV in both MCA on TCD.
Results: In 10 pts during CE and ICA clamping FV in MCA fall to „critical level" SBI (≥60%). In these group of pts hypoperfusion during CE was prevented with a temporary indwelling shunt to ensure ipsilateral hemispheric perfusion. The same group of pts was characterized by significant decrease of CVR in contralateral MCA (acetazolamide test increased FV in MCA not more than 7%), significant stenosis occlusion of contralateral ICA, disturbance of collateral functions of Circle of Willis (absence of A com A and P com A). On the other hand CVR in MCA on the side of surgery was significantly abolished in all pts and did not correlate with appearance of SBI during CE and ICA clamping.
Conclusion: The risk of SBI during CE and ICA claming correlates with preoperative assessment of disturbance of CVR in contralateral MCA, stenosis of contralateral ICA and disturbance of collateral function of Circle of Willis.

28

DUPLEX ULTRASOUND IN NEURONAVIGATION OF DEEP-SEATED CAVERNOMAS

R Stendel, A Abo Al Hassan, M Brock

Dept. of Neurosurgery, Benjamin Franklin Medical Center, Free University of Berlin, Germany

Objective: The intraoperative localization of deep-seated cavernomas may be difficult if they are small and reliable anatomical landmarks are absent. A stereotactic procedure increases the risk of the intervention and prolongs its duration. Neuronavigation may fail to detect the lesion because of brain shift. In contrast, Duplex ultrasonography combines real-time guidance with non-invasiveness.
Methods: This study includes 12 patients (mean age 36 years, range 24-52 years) with 14 cavernomas operated on using Duplex ultrasonography for intraoperative localization and monitoring of the completeness of tumor resection. The ultrasonic probes were placed directly on the cortical surface. Additional neuronavigation using the Vectorvision system (Brainlab) was performed in 4 patients.
Results: The cavernomas were located at a mean depth of 35 mm (range 5 - 65 mm) and varied in size from 5 to 15 mm (mean 9 mm). The lesions were localized using two-dimensional axial projections in all cases, and additional three-dimensional views in 4. Accompanying vessels were identified by Duplex-ultrasound in 12 of the 14 cases. Thirteen of the 14 cavernomas were successfully localized and resected using ultrasound. The one remaining lesion was a deep-seated, very small cavernoma near the crus cerebri without accompanying vessel. This lesion could not reliably be distinguished from sulci and plexus.
Conclusions: Intraoperative Duplex ultrasonography is a reliable method for real-time localization even of deep-seated small cavernomas and monitoring of their resection. Duplex ultrasound is less time consuming and less expensive than neuronavigation or intraoperative MRI. Lesions with a size of less than 6mm and deeper than 5 cm should be approached using an additional method (intraoperative MRI, stereotactic catheter placement).

29

FEEDING ARTERY DETECTION AND MONITORING OF BASAL ARTERY HEMODYNAMICS WITH COLOR-DUPLEX-SONOGRAPHY DURING SURGERY OF ARTERIOVENOUS ANGIOMAS

Woydt M, Krone A, Meixensberger J and Roosen K

Neurosurgical Department, University of Wuerzburg, Wuerzburg, Germany

Objective: With this study the potential of Colour-Duplex-Sonography (=CDS) was evaluated to detect feeding arteries and the nidus of av-angiomas and hemodynamic characteristics of basal arteries intraoperatively.

Methods: During a period of 5 years CDS was applied in 35 patients with av-angiomas (=AVM) after craniotomy and before dural closure (13 of them with power-mode). It was looked for localization of feeding arteries and the nidus, differentiation of embolized and perfused areas and the hemodynamic patterns of basal arteries during surgery.

Results: 52 out 63 angiographically verified main feeding arteries were detected by CDS by flow direction, relation to the nidus and the typical flow pattern. Additionally 3 transit arteries could be differentiated by their normal flow characteristics. Of 39 main draining veins 31 were detected. The nidus could be localized due to its characteristically dichromatic picture in 34/35 cases, embolized parts (22/22) or intracerebral haemorrhages (16/16) were identified by lack of colour-signals and typical hyperechoic appearence (haemorrhages until 10th day). In 7 patients the hemodynamic patterns of the basal arteries were followed intraoperatively: The peak systolic flow (=PSF) was stable or declined in 7/9 basal arteries (all of them at the origin of the main feeding artery), the remaining 2 showed an increased PSF (up to 30%), both of them without feeding arteries. The resistance index remained stable in 8/9 of these arteries. No "normal-perfusion-pressure-breakthrough" phenomenon was observed postoperatively in these 7 patients.

Conclusion: CDS is a non-invasive method to detect and monitor feeding and basal arteries during AVM-surgery and may be helpful to detect hemodynamic changes intraoperatively.

30

AUTIREGULATION TESTING FOR CEREBRAL ARTERIOVENOUS MALFORMATION (AVM) SURGERY.

A.L.Krivoshapkin, E.G.Melidy, V.V.Fonin, P.A.Semin, V.V.Kanygin

Novosibirsk Neurovascular Center, Russia

The surgical eradication of AVMs can be complicated by postoperative edema and hemorrhage in adjacent brain tissue, despite the total malformation excision. Various theories have been proposed to explain the hemodynamic basis for these complications, including impaired autoregulation causing "normal perfusion pressure breakthrough". Propranolol pre-treatment is recommended to prevent the complications.
The purpose of the study was to evaluate both the autoregulatory reserve capacity in AVM patients before surgery and the efficacy of Beta-blocker pre-treatment.
Twenty consecutive patients with supratentorial cerebral AVMs were examined by Transcranial Doppler (TCD) with dynamic tests for autoregulation. The transient hyperemic response test obtained by compressing the ipsilateral common carotid artery, reactivity to hypercapnia and hyperventilation were employed. According to Spetzler-Martin grades one patient had Grade I, 2 Grade II, 4 Grade III, 6 Grade IV, 7 Grade V. Fifteen patients were treated with propranolol.
The typical low peripheral resistance and high blood flow velocities in the feeding arteries were recorded in 3 Grade III, 4 Grade IV and all Grade V patients. The fully exploited autoregulatory reserve capacity was found in 12 (60%) patients. Eleven of 13 Grade IV-V patients (85%) showed impaired autoregulation. Beta blocker treatment improved the patient's autoregulatory reserve. The overshoot response recovery was observed in 8 patients (67%) on propranolol treatment in 2 weeks. There were neither pot-op normal perfusion pressure breakthrough nor new persistent neurological deficit following total AVM microsurgical excision irrespective of AVM Grades in patients with either unimpaired or recovered autoregulatory reserve capacity on propranolol pre-treatment.
The study showed the prognostic value of autoregulation testing by TCD for AVM surgery.

31

MULTIPARAMETER SENSORS AND MICRODIALYSIS MONITORING DURING ANEURYSM SURGERY: PREDICTIVE VALUE FOR INFARCTION

R Kett-White, PJ Hutchinson, P Al-Rawi, A Gupta, PJ Kirkpatrick,
Department of Neurosurgery, University of Cambridge, UK

Background: Multiparameter tissue gas sensors and microdialysis catheters have been used to monitor cerebral ischaemia in patients following acute neurological injury. This study explores the sensitivities of such parameters to well-defined periods of ischaemia accompanying aneurysm surgery, and their predictive value for infarction.
Methods and results: Neurotrend (pO_2, pCO_2, pH, temperature) sensors (Codman, USA) and microdialysis catheters (CMA, Sweden) were inserted into the vascular territory just prior to craniotomy. In 26 patients the effects of temporary vascular clamping (mean duration 16 minutes) were assessed. 3 patients subsequently declared infarction in the region of the probe. Brain pO_2 fell from a mean 3.2 (95%CI 2.4-4.1) kPa to a minimum of 1.5 (95%CI 1.0-2.0) kPa in the non-infarct group. There was a lower baseline pO_2 (mean 0.8 kPa) in the patients who infarcted. Brain pCO_2 mirrored cerebral oxygen changes, whereas brain pH did not change significantly in either group. Typical microdialysis changes associated with decreased brain oxygen included a delayed increase in lactate, a raised lactate/pyruvate ratio and an increased glutamate. These changes were not predictive of outcome.
Conclusion: Multiparameter sensors can be sensitive to acute ischaemia. Microdialysis shows potential in the assessment of metabolic changes during tissue hypoxia.

32

INVESTIGATION OF TRANSCRANIAL DOPPLER (TCD) POWER OUTPUT FOR POTENTIATION OF TISSUE PLASMINOGEN ACTIVATOR (tPA) THERAPY IN STROKE

MA Moehring, AH Voie, MP Spencer, DW Amory, AV Alexandrov

BACKGROUND: One hour 2 MHz TCD monitoring of the residual flow signals at presumed occlusion site during intravenous tPA infusion may lead to 10-15% improvement in recanalization and earlier recovery in stroke patients[1]. Literature reports suggest that ultrasound-enhanced thrombolysis increases with lower frequencies ($10\text{-}10^2$ kHz) and acoustic intensities well above 720mW/cm^2. We aimed to investigate power levels and frequencies used for clinical monitoring of tPA therapy[1].

METHODS: The study unit (Multigon 500M) was evaluated with wet tank testing using low(0-150kHz, B&K 8103) and high(.5-2.5MHz, NTR TNU100A) frequency hydrophones. The frequency response of the transducer (Spencer Technologies) was measured using an arbitrary waveform generator (LeCroy 410 Wave Station). All measurements were done at 100% diagnostic power allowed by the source unit.

RESULTS: The probe had a stop band in the frequency regime below 150kHz. In this band, signals were attenuated by >70dB relative to the center of the pass band at 2MHz. Pulse repetition frequency was found to be 10.2kHz, with 11.8mm sample volume(~30 cycles of 2MHz carrier per pulse repetition). Study monitoring was done at depths 44-58mm, and the derated spatial peak temporal average intensity (ISPTA) at 45mm depth was measured at 739mW/cm^2. The ISPTA measured in the low frequency pass band (< 150kHz) hydrophone did not exceed 1 nanoWatt/cm^2.

CONCLUSIONS: Primary power output used for tPA monitoring was at diagnostic power levels and in the vicinity of 2MHz, thereby making unlikely mechanisms of thrombolysis enhancement such as cavitation or mechanical disruption of clot. Reversible changes in fibrin structure within clot and microstreaming at the clot/blood flow boundary are hypothesized as the primary mechanisms of 2MHz potentiation of tPA lysis. A randomized clinical trial is planned.

1. AV Alexandrov, *et al*, High rate of complete recanalization and dramatic clinical recovery during tPA infusion when continuously monitored with 2-MHz transcranial Doppler monitoring, ***Stroke***, 2000;31:610-614.

33

VASOMOTOR REACTIVITY OF ANTERIOR CEREBRAL ARTERY IN PATIENTS WITH CAROTID OCCLUSIVE DISEASE

N.M. BORNSTEIN, A.Y. GUR, T. NISSEL, S. LORENZ
Stroke Unit, Department of Neurology, Tel Aviv Sourasky Medical Center, Tel Aviv, Israel

The anterior cerebral artery (ACA) may play an important role as a collateral channel in patients with internal carotid artery stenosis. Using a paired t-test we compared the cerebral vasomotor reactivity (VMR) in the ACA and middle cerebral artery (MCA) in 59 patients with unilateral severe internal carotid artery (>70%) stenosis. VMR was assessed using TCD (Rimed Intra-View) and the Diamox test. Twenty-five patients were symptomatic (SCAS) and 34 patients were asymptomatic (ACAS). The MCA VMR% on the side of carotid stenosis was found to be 34.1± 31.5% and the MCA VMR% on the opposite side was 38.8 ± 40.9% (P=0.5,NS) among the patients as a whole. The ACA VMR% on the side of carotid stenosis was 28.7 ± 35.5% and 34.5 ± 43.8% on the opposite side(P=0.3,NS). In the SCAS patients, the MCA VMR% on the side of carotid stenosis and the opposite side were 40.2 ± 40.9% and 31.3 ± 36.4%, respectively (P=0.5,NS). The ACA VMR% was 36.4 ±36.3% on the side of carotid stenosis and 33.5 ± 44.3% on the opposite side (P=0.7,NS). In the ACAS patients, the MCA VMR% on the side of carotid stenosis was 29.7 ± 21.9% and 44.3 ± 43.5% on the opposite side (P=0.08,NS). The ACA VMR% was 23 ± 34.2% and 35.3 ± 44.1% on the side of carotid stenosis and the opposite side respectively (P=0.17,NS). Our data demonstrate a similar VMR of both the ACA and MCA regardless of carotid stenosis and symptomatic or asymptomatic course of carotid occlusive disease.

34

TIME DELAY AS PARAMETER FOR CEREBROVASCULAR REACTIVITY IN PATIENTS WITH SEVERE CAROTID STENOSES

A. Hetzel, B. Guschlbauer
Department of Neurology and Neurophysiology, University of Freiburg, Germany

Background and Purpose: Responsiveness to CO_2 is an established test of cerebrovascular reserve capacity. So far only the amplitude of reaction of cerebral blood flow velocity (CBFV) and of arterial blood pressure (BP) was investigated. The aim of our study was to analyze additionally the time delay as parameter for cerebrovascular reactivity.

Methods: Sixty patients with unilateral severe carotid stenoses underwent examination defined by a protocol with multimodality monitoring of BP, pCO_2 and CBFV of both middle cerebral arteries. Beside the established CO_2 reactivity and parameters for arteriolar vasoconstriction (critical closing pressure, pulsatility index) we measured the time delay up to maximal CBFV after reaching steady-state hypercapnia and up to fall in CBFV after end of maneuver.

Results: Increase in pCO_2 was accompanied by a parallel increase of time-mean values of CBFV (ipsilateral to stenosis 1.4% / mmHg, contralateral 2.7±1.3% / mmHg CO_2). BP levels were significantly elevated during hypercapnia (time-mean values 0.9±0.5 mmHg / mmHg CO_2). Parameter of vasoconstriction showed a decrease over time on both sides, significantly lower ipsilaterally to carotid stenosis. Only the prolonged time delay at the end of hypercapnia on the side of severe obstruction reached the level of high significance (9.4±5.0 s vs. 15.6±6.6 s, $p<0.0001$)

Conclusions: Evaluation of cerebrovascular reactivity showed regarding to amplitude, time delay and parameters of active vasoconstriction significant responses to CO_2 Therefore CO_2 reactivity test should not only include the established analysis of amplitudes but also other parameters for vasomotor reactivity. Especially the time delay between fall in CO_2 and CBFV should be taken in account. For instance relevant side-to-side differences in time delay with still normal maximal increase in CBFV indicate impaired CO_2 reactivity. How far this signs of diminished autoregulatory capacity has clinical consequences has to be evaluated in our ongoing follow-up study.

35

INTRODUCTION OF A READING PARADIGM FOR NEUROVASCULAR COUPLING AND MOBILE f-TCD

B. Rosengarten, M. Kaps
Justus Liebig University at Giessen, Germany

Background and Purpose: Neurovascular coupling is a fast mechanism which adapts cerebral blood supply to cortical activity. Endothelial dysfunction is a term indicating a disturbance in this mechanism. Transcranial doppler sonography can measure neurovascular coupling but hampered flexibility because of quantification methods which needed highly standardized stimulation settings. Overcoming this need by quantificating blood flow reaction in terms of a control system we searched for a stimulation paradigm allowing maximal diagnostic flexibility. Thus we tested the reading of a newsmagazine as a visual stimulation paradigm.

Methods: We analyzed the blood flow velocity curves of the right posterior cerebral artery (PCA) stimulated by a short (20 seconds of reading) and long reading test (40 seconds of reading) in 14 healthy students and repeated both tests after some days to calculate the retest reliability. In 11 other students we performed the long reading test and analyzed the data from both PCA for side differences. Also the data of both student groups were compared.

The statistical analysis was done by a paired t- test for the original data and those obtained from the control system analyze.

Results: For stimulation- congruent phases the short and long reading test showed no significant differences in regulation of blood flow. Also between test and retest and between left and right side of the posterior cerebral artery we found no differences. Differences in the curves of both student groups are – speaking in terms of control system theory- caused by different gain values.

Conclusions: We validated an easy to perform reading test which allows a high flexibility of the doppler method. Using this paradigm in combination with quantification methods in terms of a control system even the data of different workgroups become comparable.

36

TCD CHANGES IN PATIENTS WITH AUTONOMIC NEUROPATHY

B. Žvan, M. Zaletel, T. Pogačnik
University Medical Center Ljubljana, Slovenia

Introduction: Diabetes mellitus impairs the autonomous nervous syste (ANS). This study was aimed to assess the influence of ANS on mean arterial velocity (v_m) in patients with and without evidence of ANS damage.
Methods: In 20 healthy volunteers of both genders (age 48±6.8 yrs), in 20 patients of both genders (aged 51±12 yrs) with diabetes type I or II treated with insulin and pathological findings on cardiocirculatory tests of the ANS (group A), in whom diabetes was present for 18.3 years and 20 patients of both genders (age 49±10 yrs) with type I or II diabetes treated with insulin and without laboratory evidence of ANS neuropathy (group B) and 11.8 year history of diabetes v_m was measured in both middle cerebral arteries (MCA's) with TCD. Mean arterial pressure (MAP), heart rate (HR) and Et-CO_2 were also measured. 5-min measurement of all the parameters at rest was followed by the evaluation during cold pressure test (CPT), and head-up tilt test (HUT). To analyze the value of variables we used the paired t-test, Student's t-test, ANOVA for repeated measurements, the areas beneath the ROC-curves and multi-variate analysis.
Results: There was significant difference between the two groups with respect to the duration of diabetes (p=0.00), as well as in the intensity of pain during CPT in all three groups (p=0.00). In all three groups the v_m significantly increased during CPT and decreased during HUT (p=0.00). The results of Δv_m have indicated significant differences in v_m between CPT and HUT within each individual group, as well as differences in the dynamics of v_m changes in both groups of diabetics in comparison with the healthy one (p=0.00). The model of the areas beneath the ROC-curves of v_m yielded significance so during CPT (p=0,00) as well as during HUT (p=0,00). The t-test showed differences in v_m on CPT between all three groups, while on HUT in Δv_m were observed only between group A and healthy. A multivariate analysis of CPT and HUT confirmed a significant influence of diabetes on v_m change, while MAP, HR and Et-CO_2 did not influence v_m.
Conclusions: During CPT the constriction potential in both groups of diabetics is significantly lower than in healthy population. On the other hand, during HUT the dilatation potential was found to be significantly worse only in diabetics with already proven autonomous neuropathy. It can be concluded that diabetics have less efficient cerebrovascular reactivity and thus also a narrower area of effective cerebral autoregulation activity.

37

TRANSCRANIAL DOPPLER MONITORING DURING HEAD-DOWN TILT: A TOOL TO INVESTIGATE NON-SYMPATHETIC CEREBRAL AUTOREGULATORY PATHWAY .

D. Bosone, V. Ozturk*, Roatta° S., A. Cavallini, P. Tosi, G. Micieli.
Neurovascular Unit, University of Pavia, Italy. ° Department of Human Physiology, University of Turin, Italy, *University of Dokuz Eylul, Izmir, Turkiye.

Background: It is accepted that the sympathetic system exerts a protective role of cerebral tissue in chronic hypertensive conditions, while its role in vascular auto-regulation of normotensive subjects is still matter of controversy. In the present work we aim at investigating hemodynamic changes induced by Head Down Tilt, an experimental model which can produce acute hypertensive state at the cranial level, inducing a reflex sympathetic inhibition.
Methods: A total 20 healthy volunteers aged 20-41 years were studied for 10 minutes during basal supine position , during 30° head-down (HDT) tilt position and during basal supine position again. Blood flow velocities (CBV) from middle cerebral artery were continuously monitored with TCD, as were mean arterial blood pressure (MAP) and heart rate (HR) using a non-invasive finger-cuff method.
Results: Compared with the basal supine position: MAP slightly decreased during HDT and recovery; HR increased a little more than basal value at the beginning of the test, decreasing in the late phase of HDT; CBV increased for all the tilt duration; PI also increased during the first minute of HDT, then decreasing gradually toward basal values, while the ratio MAP/CBV sharply decreased at the beginning of the HDT.
Conclusions: Our results support the global inhibition of the sympathetic activity induced by HDT in normotensive subjects. We disagree with previous TCD studies, reporting increase in blood flow and autoregulatory increase in vascular resistances; considering the evidence of a reduction of cerebral perfusion pressure during HDT, we suggest that the CBV increase could be due to a small decrease in the MCA diameter and that resistances are reduced as the effect of the autoregulatory mechanism facing a reduced perfusion pressure.

38

CEREBRAL HAEMODYNAMICS DURING VASOVAGAL SYNCOPE

BJ Carey, PJ Eames, RB Panerai and JF Potter
Division of Medicine for the Elderly, University of Leicester, Glenfield Hospital, Leicester, UK.

Introduction
It is unclear whether cerebral autoregulation (CA) is impaired prior to vasovagal syncope (VVS) with both paradoxical increases and appropriate decreases in cerebrovascular resistance (CVR) being reported. Critical closing pressure (CrCP) refers to the pressure below which blood flow in a vessel ceases. Resistance-area product (RAP) is an index of cerebrovascular resistance (CVR) that takes CrCP into account. This study clarifies the cerebral haemodynamics of VVS using CrCP and RAP.
Methods
15 patients with recurrent VVS and 65 normal subjects were subjected to 30 minutes of 70° head-up tilt. Bilateral middle cerebral artery (MCA) blood flow velocities (CBFV) were measured using transcranial Doppler ultrasound and MCA pressure estimated by using the Finapres device at heart level and adjusting values for height. Heart rate and end-tidal and transcutaneous carbon dioxide (CO_2) levels were monitored simultaneously.
Results
All 15 patients and 13 normal subjects developed VVS. During pre-syncope, mean CBFV declined in tandem with the decline in MCA pressure but diastolic CBFV declined to a greater extent than systolic CBFV (49% v 7%, p<0.001). CO_2 levels and RAP decreased during pre-syncope while CrCP increased, approaching MCA diastolic pressure, before decreasing precipitously on syncope. All changes in the pre-syncopal period were similar for patients and normal subjects.
Conclusions
The fall in CBFV suggests that CA is impaired during pre-syncope despite a fall in RAP and, hence, CVR. The rise in CrCP during pre-syncope is probably due to hypocapnia and accounts for the selective fall in diastolic CBFV. Rises in CrCP, therefore, offset falls in CVR leading to impaired CA prior to VVS.

39

CEREBRAL BLOOD FLOW VELOCITY (CBFV) DURING UPRIGHT TILT IN CHRONIC FATIGUE SYNDROME (CFS)

A Razumovsky, K DeBusk, H Calkins, S Snader, P Vyas, D Hanley, PC Rowe. Johns Hopkins Medical Institutions, Baltimore, USA

Background: During head-up tilt (HUT), patients with CFS have higher rates of neurally mediated hypotension (NMH) and tachycardia. We studied whether these changes were associated with abnormal CBFV. **Methods:** Transcranial Doppler (TCD) monitoring of middle cerebral artery (MCA) mean CBFV was performed during 3-stage HUT (method described in *JAMA 1995;274:961-7*) prospectively in 26 subjects with CFS (23 F, mean age 33.6 yrs) and 23 healthy controls (18 F; mean age 29.9 yrs). Results are reported as mean±SD. **Results:** NMH developed in 21/26 with CFS and in 14/23 controls (P=0.22). Supine HR was higher in CFS patients 76.1±12.1 vs 62.4±8.1 (P < 0.001) but all other hemodynamic and CBFV variables were similar at baseline. Patients with CFS had a higher peak HR in the first 10 min and in the first 45 min of upright tilt (P<0.01). The median time to hypotension did not differ, but the median time to onset of orthostatic symptoms was shorter in those with CFS (10 min vs. 26 min; P < 0.001). Systolic, diastolic, and mean CBFV did not differ between groups in the supine posture, but pulsatility index (PI) was lower in those with CFS (0.51±0.1 vs 0.57±0.1 (P=0.04). CBFV did not differ between groups at 1- or 5-minutes after upright tilt, or at 5- or 1-minute before the end of the test, or at termination of the test. CBFV fell from 66.2±17.4 cm/sec supine to 31.8±15.4 cm/sec at termination of tilt testing in those with CFS, vs 74.0±13.2 cm/sec supine to 39.0±17.1 cm/sec in controls (P=0.13). End-tidal CO2 was lower at termination of the test in those with CFS (N=16) vs controls (N=21): 23.2±6.5 mmHg vs 30.8 ±7.1 mmHg (P=0.002). **Conclusions:** Patients with CFS and healthy controls had similar rates of orthostatic intolerance during HUT, and similar changes in CBFV. Our data are not consistent with the hypothesis that those with CFS have a distinctive pattern of CBFV changes in response to orthostatic stress.

40

B- AND M-WAVES IN VARIOUS TYPES OF HEADACHE

U Sliwka, S Harscher, R v. Schayck, CC Eschenfelder, C Weiller
Friedrich-Schiller-University, Dept. of Neurology, Jena, Germany

Background and Purpose: B- and Mayer (M)-waves are spontaneous oscillations in cerebral blood flow velocity (CBFV) with frequency of 0.5-3 or 4-7 cycles per minute (cpm), respectively, measured by transcranial Doppler (TCD). There is evidence that B-waves are generated by certain brain stem nuclei, which modulate the lumen of the small intracerebral vessels via monoaminergic nerve endings. In contrast, M-waves in CBFV mirror the M-waves in arterial blood pressure and represent peripheral autonomic activity. Migraine may be generated by a neurotransmitter dysbalance in the brain stem nuclei. Impairment of the peripheral autonomic nervous system was observed in patients with chronic tension headache (CTH). Hypothesis: 1. Migraine patients have B-wave abnormalities in comparison to normal controls or CTH patients. 2. CTH patients have an imbalance in autonomic activity which will be reflected in differences of M-wave activity in comparison to normal controls.
Methods: B- and M-waves were studied in 30 patients with migraine without aura, 28 subjects with CTH and 30 normal controls using bilateral TCD monitoring of the middle cerebral artery (MCA) for 15 minutes each. Coefficient of variation (CoV) as a quantitative parameter for amplitude of waves and the mean frequency were calculated from the envelope curves of the Doppler spectra.
Results: CoV of B-waves was higher in migraine patients compared to patients with CTH or normal controls ($p<0.05$). Patients with CTH had lower CoV-values for M-wave activity in comparison to normal controls ($p<0.05$).
Conclusions: Our data support the hypothesis of dysfunction of the brain stem monoaminergic/serotonergic system in migraine. In contrast, patients with CTH have decreased sympathetic activity.

41

HARMONIC IMAGING OF THE BASAL CEREBRAL ARTERIES

S. Horner (*), M. Augustin (*), G. Bone (*), E. Klein (**),
R. Schmidt (*), T. Schober (*), K. Niederkorn (*).
Dep. of Neurology (*) and Dep. of Radiology (**), Karl Franzens University, Graz, Austria.
fax +43 316 385 3512
e-mail: susanna.horner@kfunigraz.ac.at

Objective: Diameter measurement is a prerequisite for flow volume calculation by transcranial color-coded Duplex sonography (TCCD). This study aimed to determine the reliability of different ultrasound modes in establishing middle cerebral artery (MCA) diameter when digital subtraction angiography (DSA) is used as gold standard. Magnetic resonance angiography (MRA) was additionally performed.
Methods: The diameters of 42 non-stenotic MCA´s, measured at 5 mm distance of the MCA origin, were calculated from DSA and MRA images. Mean values were compared with TCCD (Vingmed, Norway) calculations, obtained by different Doppler modes, including color Doppler (CD), power Doppler (PD), harmonic imaging (HI), contrast color Doppler (cCD) and contrast power Doppler (cPD). Contrast studies were performed by repeated intravenous injection of (1 ml per vessel side) Optison® (Mallinckrodt Medical GmbH, Germany), an albumin-based suspension with defined properties.
Results: The mean MCA diameter (mm) was 2.2 ± 0.4 and 2.2 ± 0.2 as assessed by DSA and MRA, respectively. The values of CD, PD, **HI**, cCD and cPD were: 3.7 ±0.8, 4.4 ± 1.3, **2.7** ± 0.5, 4.4 ± 1.0 and 4.6 ±1.0.
Conclusion: All ultrasound methods overestimated the MCA diameter. HI revealed the most accurate results. These data suggest HI to be best suited for ultrasound-based intracranial vessel measurements.

42

Comparison of Pulse Inversion Contrast Harmonic Imaging and Xenon-CT in Evaluation of Brain Perfusion

S. Meairs, P. Horn*, R. Kern, J. Beyer, P. Schmiedek*, M. Hennerici
Departments of Neurology and Neurosurgery*, University of Heidelberg, Klinikum Mannheim, 68135 Mannheim, Germany

Purpose: Pulse inversion contrast harmonic imaging (PICHI) is a promising new technique for assessment of brain perfusion. We sought to further characterize this method by comparing bolus wash-out curves with flow measurements obtained by Xenon-CT.
Methods: Seven patients were examined after extracranial bypass surgery. All patients had ipsilateral ICA occlusions and had suffered from transient ischemic attacks due to poor collateralization. PICHI was performed with an HDI 5000 (ATL) using a 2-5 MHz dynamic range curved array transducer, which was mounted upon a stand to eliminate probe movement. Insonation was through the trepanation defect. A bolus of Levovist® (Schering AG) (3.6 g, 300 mg/dl) was infused at 3 ml/sec with a Pulsar Ultrasound Injection System® (Medrad). Intermittent imaging was performed every 3 seconds with a mechanical index of 0.9. Contrast enhancement was measured in 10 mm^2 regions of interest positioned symmetrically in both temporal lobes using HDILab©. Xeon-CT (DDP Inc.) was done on a GE Pace scanner with a 4.5 min wash-in protocol using 30% Xenon and 60% O_2. The β fit parameter of contrast wash-out was compared to Xenon-CT measurements of mean flow in the temporal lobes.
Results: Ipsilateral mean flow with Xenon-CT ranged from 25-48 m/min (mean 43 ml/min, SD ± 11 ml/min). The β fit parameter of PICHI wash-out ranged from 0.06-0.14 (mean 0.11 ± 0.03) The correlation of mean flow values with the β fit parameter of PICHI washout was r=0.82.
Conclusions: The results of this study indicate that the β fit parameter of PICHI bolus wash-out curves can provide meaningful information on brain perfusion.

43

ASSESSMENT OF CEREBRAL PERFUSION RESERVE WITH SECOND HARMONIC IMAGING

J. Federlein, E. Karagiannis, S. Meves, Th. Büttner H. Przuntek, Th. Postert
Department of Neurology, Ruhr-University Bochum, Germany

Introduction: Second harmonic imaging (SHI) enables visualization of parenchymal cerebral echo contrast enhancement in different brain areas. Aim of the present study was to evaluate and compare quantitative parameters in SHI examinations prior to and after application of azetazolamide in healthy individuals and patients with internal carotid artery occlusion.
Methods: SHI (after application of 4 g galactose-based microbubbles) and transcranial color-coded real-time examinations were performed in 6 healthy volunteers (mean age 34,6 years) and 3 patients (mean age 64,8 years) with asymptomatic occlusion of the internal carotid artery. Mean middle cerebral artery flow velocities were measured in TCCS examinations. PIs and AUCs were calculated off-line in the region of the lentiform nucleus and the white matter. All examinations and calculations were repeated after intravenous injection of 1 g acetazolamide.
Results: In all volunteers and patients an increase of the mean flow velocity of the MCA could be observed after application of acetazolamide indicating preserved cerebrovascular reserve capacity. Mean increase of PIs and AUCs in SHI examinations of the white matter was 29 and 26,5%. Corresponding values for the Pis and AUCs of the lentiform nucleus were 91,6 and 107,6%, respectively.
Conclusions: Evaluation of quantitative parameters of SHI examinations after application of acetazolamide is useful for the assessment of increased parenchymal cerebral echo contrast enhancement due to vasodilatation.

44

COMPARATIVE VISUALIZATION OF BRAIN TISSUE PERFUSION IN VARIOUS NEUROLOGICAL DISORDERS UTILIZING CONTRAST-ENHANCED HARMONIC IMAGING IN INTEGRATED BACKSCATTER AND POWER DOPPLER METHODS

T. Shiogai, C. Tsunezuka, M. Koshimura, N. Takayasu [1], Y. Nagakane [1], T. Nakase [1], M. Makino[1], K. Nakajima[1], H. Furuhata [2], Department of Clinical Neurosciences, Kyoto Takeda Hospital, Department of Neurology, Kyoto Prefectural University of Medicine[1], Kyoto; ME Lab, Tokyo Jikei University School of Medicine[2], Tokyo; Japan

Objective The evaluation of brain tissue perfusion utilizing contrast-enhanced harmonic imaging (CHI) has been clinically introduced. We investigated the CHI to determine whether gray-scale imaging created by integrated backscatter (IBS) or power Doppler imaging (PDI) resulted in optimal visualization of brain tissue contrast effects with respect to patients with various neurological disorders.

Patients and Methods The subjects were 28 patients (cerebral ischemia 15, Parkinsonism 4, anoxic encephalopathy1, chronic subdural hematoma 1, hydrocephalus 1, cerebral hemorrhage 1, malignant lymphoma 1, others 4; ages 40-90, mean 72). Utilizing a color duplex ultrasound system (HP5500) with a 1.8/3.6-MHz harmonic sector transducer, transient response harmonic imagings (every 2-4 heartbeats) created by IBS and PDI after 7 ml bolus injections of contrast agent (Levovist[R], 300mg/ml) were evaluated at the level of lateral (anterior horn) and third ventricles via temporal windows. Both images (n = 55) were compared bilaterally (n=24) or unilaterally (n=7), in one or two (two cases) examinations. Contrast effects in brain tissue and vessels were evaluated on the basis of size and intensity, location, and demarcation (three visualization grade: ++, +, -).

Results 1) Contrast effects were identified in all but one image (98%) in IBS and 84% of images (n = 46) in PDI. 2) Visualization grade of IBS was superior to PDI (++: IBS 53%, PDI 24%). 3) Contrast effects in medial temporal lobe and basal ganglia were more obvious in IBS than PDI. However, PDI demonstrated extra- and intra-parenchymal vessels simultaneously. 4) Demarcation of contrast-enhanced areas was more easily identified in PDI rather than IBS.

Conclusions In evaluation of brain tissue perfusion utilizing CHI, visualization of contrast effects was more sensitive in gray-scale IBS imaging than PDI. However, it is necessary to introduce new methodologies, such as subtraction, to visualize defined contrast-enhanced areas.

45

Continuous Measurement of Contrast Induced Signal Enhancement in Transcranial Doppler Examination – a Novel Method of Quantitative R/L-Shuntvolume Assessment

JJ Schwarze[1], D Sander[2], J Klingelhöfer[1]
Department of Neurology, Chemnitz Medical Center[1] and Technical University Munich[2], Germany

Background: Paradoxical embolism through an interatrial right-to-left-shunt (RLS) is a potential cause of cerebral ischemia. More recently, have taken interest in the size of the opening and the amount of the shuntvolume is of paramount importance, as it seems to determine the clinical relevance of the RLS. However, counting the high intensity transient signals (HITS) on contrast-TCD is time consuming, and may not always be sufficiently accurate. Measuring the maximum distance between the septum primum and secundum (D_{sept}) on transesophageal echocardiography (TEE) is frequently not feasible, and disregards the shuntvolume. The present study was designed to evaluate a newly designed software program which permits a continuous quantitative analysis of the TCD signal enhancement due to ultrasonic contrast medium (CM) as a measure for the shuntvolume.

Methods: A total of 9 patients [5 male; mean age 58.7 ± 9.4 years], who had sustained a cerebrovascular accident and who had evidence for a R/L-shunt on contrast-TCD were included. The presence of a R/L-shunt was confirmed and D_{sept} was measured by a cardiologist, who was blinded to the results of the contrast-TCD examination. The software program calculated the mean intensity for every sample of the TCD spectrum. The intensity of the background signal was determined as baseline intensity, and all intensity increases above this background signal after the injection of the CM were measured and added over time. The plateau of the intensity increase thus obtained (Σ_{II}) was determined and compared to the number of HITS and D_{sept}.

Results: The average Σ_{II} was 14.1 x 10^2 dB (range 1.5–35.5 x 10^2 dB). A mean CM-HITS count of 17.4 and a mean D_{sept} of 0.67 mm was found for all 9 recordings. Both parameters, the CM-HITS count and D_{sept} correlated well with Σ_{SE}, (r=0.76, p<0.05; r=0.68, p<0.05).

Conclusion: Σ_{SE} may be a useful measure to determine the right-to-left shuntvolume and thereby the clinical relevance of the R/L-shunt. The software program is a useful tool to facilitate the off-line analysis, especially if large quantities of CM traverse the interatrial septum.

46

Indication and diagnostic benefit of the ultrasound contrast agent Levovist® in the transcranial ultrasound.

P. Zunker[1], H. Wilms[1], G. Wasner[1], A. Allardt[1], J.A. Zeller[1], J. Neumann[2], G. Deuschl[1]. Dep. of Neurology[1], Kiel University Hospital, Niemannsweg 147, 24105 Kiel, Schering Deutschland GmbH[2], Max-Dohrn-Str.10, 10589 Berlin, Germany

The application of ultrasound contrast agents (UCA) enabled the evaluation of intracranial vessels which were poorly or not at all insonable before. In this prospective study we examined a) the indication for application and b) the diagnostic benefit of the UCA Levovist in transcranial ultrasound examinations.
From July until December all patients subjected to a transcranial ultrasound examination were recruited. Indication for application of Levovist was an unsufficient diagnostic evaluation of the intracranial vessels using the transtemporal or suboccipital approach by means of transcranial Doppler or colour-coded Duplex sonography. Levovist was always given intravenously in a concentration of 300mg/ml. Effectiveness of the UCA was classified as diagnostic, improved, not improved.
687 patients were included in the study. In 61 patients (8.8%) indication for the UCA was seen, in 57 patients (8.3%) UCA was actually given. In 39 cases we studied effectiveness through the transtemporal and in 19 cases by the suboccipital approach. By the transtemporal insonation UCA in one case was without benefit. In the remaining 38 patients 112 arteries could be additionally evaluated. In 86 (76.8%) arteries the benefit was diagnostic, in 26 (23.2%) insonation was improved. Through the suboccipital approach after UCA, 31 arteries could be insonated additionally. In 25 (80.6%) arteries the benfit was diagnostic, in 6 (19.4%) signal quality had improved.
In this prospective transcranial ultrasound study indication for application of UCA (Levovist) was given in 9% of patients. Application of Levovist led to a diagnostic result of the ultrasound examination that could not be achieved without UCA in 75-80%.

47

BENEFIT OF THE ULTRASOUND CONTRAST ENHANCING AGENT LEVOVIST® IN PATIENTS WITH INSUFFICIENT TEMPORAL BONE WINDOW INVESTIGATED BY TRANSCRANIAL DOPPLER ULTRASOUND

T Hansberg[1,2], KS L Wong[1], MA Ritter[2], DW Droste[2], EB Ringelstein[2], R Kay[1]
(1=Department of Medicine and Therapeutics, Section Neurology, Prince of Wales Hospital, The Chinese University of Hong Kong; 2=Department of Neurology, University of Münster, Germany)

Background: Proper assessment of intracranial arteries by transcranial Doppler sonography (TCD) in patients with intracranial stenoses is occasionally made difficult by an insufficient temporal bone window, an unfavourable insonation angle, or low flow velocity or volume. In these cases, echocontrast could be helpful.

Methods: We investigated 48 temporal windows of 24 acute stroke patients with insufficient native transtemporal insonation conditions before and after the application of the echo-enhancer Levovist® by an injection pump. We classified the signal quality from four segments of the main intracranial arteries, anterior cerebral artery (A1), mainstem of the middle cerebral artery (M1), intracranial segment of the carotid artery (C1), posterior cerebral artery (P1). The signal quality was classified as follows: 0 = no signal, 1 = poor, envelope curve does not follow spectrum, 2 = adequate, envelope curve follows spectrum.

Results: As compared to the pre-contrast scans, echocontrast allowed for more segments to be evaluated by pulsed Doppler sonography. Before Levovist®, only 12% of the segments could be visualized, after Levovist® 63%. For all arteries, signal quality was better after Levovist®, p between .018 and .0003. In three patients, MCA stenoses with peak systolic Doppler flow velocities above 160 cm/s were found after Levovist®.

Conclusion: In patients with poor pre-contrast visualization of arteries, echocontrast-enhanced TCD can be helpful in the assessment of intracranial arteries.

48

IMPROVED IMAGING QUALITY OF INTRACRANIAL VERTEBROBASILAR ARTERIES BY CONTRAST - ENHANCED COLOUR DUPLEX

B.Iglseder, **W.Staffen, M.Huemer, G.Ladurner**

Background: Conventional transcranial colour real time sonography of the vertebrobasilar system is limited by imaging problems of the distal segment of the basilar artery. Lung stable contrast enhancing agents may overcome this problem by enhancing the quality of Doppler signals up to 20%.

Subjects and methods: 20 persons underwent sonographic evaluation of the vertebrobasilar system before and after intravenously administered albumin based contrast enhancing agent Optison™ by transforaminal and transtemporal routes. The length of visible colour flow delineated from the the basilar artery before and after Optison™ was classified into five categories and compared to the length measured by intracranial MRA.

Results: Application of intravenously administered Optison™ improves imaging quality of the basilar artery to an extent that allows nearly full coverage of all the anatomic length as compared to intracranial MRA.

Conclusions: Contrast enhanced intracranial colour duplex is a reliable tool for investigation of intracranial vertebrobasilar arteries.

Landesklinik für Neurologie
Christian Doppler Klinik (Landesnervenklinik)
Ignaz-Harrerstrasse 79, A-5020 Salzburg, Austria

49

Acceleration of thrombolysis in vivo by transcranial ultrasonication

Toshihiro Ishibashi[1], Masahiko Akiyama[1], Hisashi Onoue[1], Toshiaki Abe[1], Hiroshi Furuhata[2]
Department of Neurosurgery[1], Medical Engineering Laboratory[2], The Jikei University School of Medicine,
Tokyo Japan

[Background and Purpose]

Acceleration of thrombolysis by transcranial ultrasonication (TU) has not been previously reported in in-vivo experiments. We verified TU effects on thrombolysis in a rabbit femoral artery occlusion model using aged thrombi.

[Methods]

Thrombus Preparation: Arterial blood was drawn from rabbits auricular artery to polyethylene tubing and leave in a room temperature during 2 hours and subsequently retained for 22hours at 4℃. Procedure: New Zealand white rabbits were anesthetized and maintained with 1 1.5% isoflurane. Thrombus was left in a femoral artery under microscopic operation. Femoral artery occlusion was induced in 12 cases. Immediately after confirmation of stable occlusion, rabbits were received 0.4mg/kg a bolus of recombinant tissue plasminogen activator (t-PA). In 6 cases, ultrasound irradiates through a piece of cadaver temporal bone (4mm thickness) to the occlusion vessels. Ultrasound frequency and intensity were 212kHz and 0.142W/cm2. Ultrasound intensity through the skull was 0.016W/cm2.

[Result]

Initial recanalization was achieved in four of 6 cases (66%) with t-PA and TU, and three of 6 cases (50%) with t-PA alone respectively. The mean initial recanalization time was 20min. in t-PA and TU group, while at 38min.in t-PA alone.

[Conclusion]

It was suggested that the acceleration of thrombolysis by TU had an advantage in early recanalization of ischemic cerebral vascular disease caused by aged thrombi.

50

NON-INVASIVE MONITORING OF INTRACRANIAL PRESSURE AND COMPLIANCE

K. Paulat, R. Brucher, D. Russell. Ulm University of Applied Sciences, Germany and Dept of Neurology, The National Hospital, Oslo, Norway.

Introduction: The quality of the management of patients with intracranial disease is greatly improved if intracranial pressure (ICP) and pressure/volume relationships i.e. compliance/elastance may be continuously monitored. At present, however, this may only be achieved invasively which carries a considerable risk for serious complications.

Methods and results: In this study we demonstrate the feasibility of a new non-invasive method for measuring ICP and compliance in 10 healthy controls. ICP variations were assessed by measuring tympanic membrane ICP propagation. This is possible since ICP and its infrasonic pressure waves are transmitted through the aquaeductus chochleae and the middle ear towards the tympanic membrane. The middle ear and the tympanic membrane act as a pressure transformer. Movement of the tympanic membrane results in pressure fluctuations in the outer ear channel which are measured using a specially designed pressure transducer. Changes in ICP during monitoring cause therefore corresponding changes in the pressure transducer. Attenuation factors are subject dependant which requires calibration of the system at two different venous hydrostatic pressures. Cerebral compliance was measured by simultaneously assessing the Windkessel volume displacement of the cerebral arteries (1). This is achieved by measuring the cross-section TCD power index with corrections for the Doppler frequency distributions (frequency corrected power).

Conclusion: We have demonstrated that it is now possible to non-invasively monitor intracranial pressure and compliance. This new method should now be assessed in more extensive clinical studies.

Reference

1. Paulat K, Brucher R, Russell D. Non-invasive assessment of intracranial compliance. Cerebrovasc Dis 1999; (suppl 2):55.

51

CONTRAST AGENT SPECIFIC IMAGING MODES FOR THE ULTRASONIC ASSESSMENT OF BRAIN PERFUSION

Th. Postert, P. Hoppe, J. Federlein, S. Helbeck*, H. Ermert*, H. Przuntek, Th. Büttner, W. Wilkening*
Department of Neurology, Department of Electrical Engineering, Ruhr-University Bochum, Germany*

Our study was designed to explore possible advantages of two new contrast agent specific imaging modes, contrast burst (CBI) and time variance imaging (TVI) that are based on the detection of destruction or splitting of microbubbles caused by ultrasound, in comparison to contrast harmonic imaging.

Subjects and Methods: CHI, CBI and TVI examinations were performed in 9 healthy individuals after an intravenous bolus injection of 4 g galactose-based microbubble suspension. Using time-intensity curves, peak intensities (PIs) and times to peak intensities (TPIs) were calculated off-line in anterior and posterior parts of the thalamus, in the lentiform nucleus, and in the white matter. The potential of the different techniques to visualize cerebral contrast enhancement in different brain areas was compared.

Results: All techniques produced accurate cerebral contrast enhancement in the majority of investigated brain areas. CHI visualized in 28 out of 36 ROIs signal increase after application of Levovist. In comparison, TVI and CBI examinations were successful in 32 and 35 investigations, respectively. In CHI examinations contrast enhancement was most difficult to visualize in posterior parts of the thalamus (6/9) and the lentiform nucleus (6/9). For all investigated imaging modes, PIs and TPIs in different ROIs did not differ significantly, except that TVI demonstrated significantly higher Pis in the lentiform nucleus as compared to the thalamus and the white matter ($p<0.05$).

Conclusions: The present study demonstrates for the first time that CBI and TVI represent new ultrasonic tools that allow noninvasive assessment of focal cerebral contrast enhancement and that CBI and TVI improve diagnostic sensitivity as compared to CHI.

52

SONOGRAPHIC BRAIN TUMOR IMAGING USING STIMULATED ACOUSTIC EMISSION

M. Lange, B. Draganski, F. Schlachetzki,
T. Hölscher, L. Kouznetsova, U. Bogdahn
Klinik Universität Regensburg, Regensburg, Germany

Background and Objectives: Transcranial colour coded sonography (TCCS) is an additional tool in assessing brain tumor morphology and vascularisation. Stimulated acoustic emission (SAE) -imaging with ultrasound contrast agents (UCA) may be used to study brain tumor perfusion and thus to assess tumor malignancy and treatment response. In this pilot-study we tested the efficacy of the albumin based perfluorgas FS O69 in SAE-perfusion imaging in brain tumors.

Methods: Six patients with primary intracerebral tumors were examined before and after bolus-application of FS O69. Perfusion as detected by SAE-imaging technique was correlated to HMPAO-SPECT and diffusion weighted MRI (DWI). Contrast enhancement was compared between the tumor-affected hemisphere and the corresponding healthy tissue of the contalateral side.

Results: Using DWI and HMPAO-SPECT perfusion in tumor tissue was visualized. Employing SAE time-intensity-curves were generated with the region of interest (ROI) placed in the suspected tumor area. We could demonstrate that low grade braintumors as well as high grade glioblastomas have a different perfusion when compared to normal tissue.

Conclusions: Our results indicate that SAE may be useful in assessing tumor perfusion in selected patients. Moreover perfusion differences as seen in SAE-imagung are comparable to DWI and HMPAO-SPECT in patients with intracerebral tumors.
Further studies are needed to investigate the sensitivity of sonographic diagnosis of intracerebral neoplasms and quantifying its perfusion by the use of UCAs.

53

VOLUME FLOW CHANGES IN THE VERTEBRAL VEINS DURING BILATERAL INTERNAL JUGULAR VEIN AND CIRCULAR NECK COMPRESSION

J.M. Valdueza, F. Lürtzing, S.J. Schreiber, K.M. Einhäupl
Dept. of Neurology, University Hospital Charité, Berlin, Germany

Objective: To assess the significance of extrajugular cerebral outflow pathways in the neck.
Methods: Volume flow measurements of the internal jugular veins (IJVs) and vertebral veins (VVs) were performed at rest in 12 healthy young volunteers using duplex sonography. Measurements were repeated in the VVs during transient bilateral IJV occlusion and circular neck compression. Complete obstruction of flow in the IJVs was confirmed by duplex sonography. Circular neck compression was achieved by an elastic band. An additional obstruction of deep neck veins was assumed.
Results: Total venous flow volume was 766±226 ml/min at rest. The IJVs contributed 94% (720±223 ml/min) and both VVs 6% (46±32 ml/min). Volume flow increased in the VVs during bilateral IJV occlusion to 128±61 ml/min (18% of total outflow). A further increase to 183±69 ml/min (26% of total outflow) was noted during circular neck compression.
Conclusions: 1. The results give further evidence that the VVs are important collateral venous pathways for the brain. 2. The contribution of the deep neck veins in the drainage of the cerebral blood in bilateral IJV occlusion is limited. 3. The flow increase in the VVs is not sufficient to compensate for the cessation in jugular flow. It seems that the intraspinal venous plexus has to be considered as the main alternative drainage pathway.

54

Reproducibility of Three-Dimensional (3-D) Ultrasound Regarding the Depiction of Carotid Artery Plaque Ulceration

U. Schminke, L. Motsch, C. Kessler
Department of Neurology, University of Greifswald, Germany

Carotid artery plaque ulceration has been shown to be associated with an increased risk of cerebral embolism. However, there is still controversy about the ability of conventional 2-D ultrasound and angiography (DSA) to identify ulcerated plaques. The recently developed 3-D ultrasound technique facilitates visualization of the luminal plaque surface. The present study was designed to assess the repeatability of 3-D ultrasound for the depiction of carotid artery plaque ulceration.
3-D ultrasound examinations of 17 carotid artery plaques with an ulcerated surface according to 2-D duplex ultrasound criteria were performed in a prospective study with 16 patients (10 male; 6 female; mean age 68.9 ± 7.1 yr.). Acquisition of exactly parallel B-mode ultrasound scans (slice distance 0.1mm) was performed using a 5 MHz linear array probe (G.E. Diasonics, Milpitas, Ca) clamped in a probe carriage device and propelled by a mechanical step motor. The recorded images were reconstructed to a volumetric data set in a Cartesian coordinate system (TOMTEC Echoscan, Munich, Germany). The data sets were reviewed by two independent observers who were blinded to the results of each other and repeated by one of them at different days. After plaque segmentation and 3-D reconstruction of the luminal plaque surface the diameter of the 3-D displayed ulceration was determined. The agreement between two readings was evaluated using Bland-Altman analysis.
The mean diameter of the plaque ulceration was 2.3 ± 1.1 mm (1. observer) and 2.4 ± 1.2 mm (2. observer), respectively. The limits of intraobserver agreement (mean ± 2 SD) ranged from -0.21 to 0.22 mm (–8.9% to 9.4%) and the limits of interobserver agreement ranged from -0.23 to 0.05 mm (-9.7% to 2.3%).
In conclusion, the present study has shown an excellent repeatability for 3-D display of plaque ulceration comparable to the results of previous 3-D ultrasound studies assessing the reproducibility of plaque volume measurement.

55

DETECTION OF THE ANTERIOR AND POSTERIOR COMMUNICATING ARTERY USING 3D-TRANSCRANIAL COLOR-CODED DUPLEXSONOGRAPHY

[1]Christof Klötzsch, [1]R.Caspary, [1]G.Lammers, [2]M.Mull, [1]J.Noth
Dept.of [1]Neurology and [2]Neuroradiology, RWTH Aachen, Germany

Background: The role of two-dimensional transcranial color-coded sonography (2D-TCCS) as a diagnostic tool in cases of vascular alteration is unquestioned. The detection of intracranial collaterals, however, may be a difficult task. The clinical value of a personal computer-based, 3D-reconstruction system for TCCS was used to demonstrate the anterior and posterior communicating artery (AcomA, PcomA).
Methods: 83 consecutive patients were enrolled in the study (39 men, 44 women; mean age: 54±14 years). The TCCS examinations were performed with a 2-MHz probe using the power mode. The 3D-system (3D-Echotech®, Germany) consisted of an electromagnet, which induced a low-intensity magnetic field. A magnetic position sensor was attached to the ultrasound probe and transmitted the spatial orientation to a computer, which also received the corresponding 2D-images from the duplex machine. The echo contrast enhancer D-galactose (Levovist®, Schering, Germany) was used in all patients to improve the signal-to-noise ratio. The decision to perform digital subtraction angiography (DSA) was made on a clinical basis to investigate extra- or intracranial vessel disease.
Results: In 59 of 83 patients (60%) it was possible to demonstrate the AcomA using 3D-TCCS. The precommunicating segment of the anterior cerebral artery was visible in 111 of 166 cases (67%). The PcomA was shown in 113 of 166 cases (68%), one vessel revealed duplication. In 6 patients an embryonal origin of the posterior cerebral artery was observed. Insufficient correlation with angiographic results was caused by bad insonation conditions (58%) and hypoplastic vessels (42%).
Conclusions: Using 3D-TCCS, the inconstant insonation conditions in consecutive patients make the differentiation between aplasia and insufficient detection of small and short collateral vessels difficult. In patients with sufficient bone windows it is usually possible to demonstrate anatomic variations like duplications or aplasia of collateral vessels.

56

Patent Foramen Ovale and Internal Jugular Valve Incompetence in Transient Global Amnesia: A Contrast Transcranial Doppler Sonography and Color Flow Imaging of Internal Jugular Vein

Maalikjy Akkawi N., Agosti C., Anzola G.P., Morandi E., Vignolo L.A., Zavarise P., Padovani A.
Clinica Neurologica Università di Brescia
Brescia - Italy

Objective: Valsalvalike activities often precede the onset of transient global amnesia (TGA). The pathogenesis of TGA is still unknown. Both paradoxical embolism due to a patent foramen ovale and venous cerebral ischemia due to internal jugular valve incompetence (IJVI) have been proposed as causative factors. We have investigated the frequency of patent foramen ovale (PFO) and the internal jugular valve competence in patients with TGA compared to age matched patients with transient ischemic attack (TIA).

Design: Consecutive patients assessed for either TGA or TIA at the Neurological Unit, Department of Medical Science, Spedali Civili, Brescia, Italy. PFO was examined by contrast transcranial Doppler sonography. Internal jugular valve competence was checked by color flow and spectral imaging.

Patients: 30 patients with TGA were compared to 20 aged matched patients with TIA.

Results: PFO was found in 20% (6/30) of patients with TGA and in 25% (5/20) of the control group with TIA. Inversion of the jugular vein flow during the Valsalva Maneuver was observed in 40% (12/30) of patients with TGA and in 30% (6/20) of the control group with TIA. There was no significant difference between the two groups in the frequency of PFO and IJVI.

Conclusions: this preliminary study failed to demonstrate differences between TGA and TIA patients with regard to PFO and IJVI. These findings argue against the hypothesis that paradoxical embolism plays a fundamental role in TGA. Data in venous cerebral ischemia require further investigations.

57

HYPERDENSE MIDDLE CEREBRAL ARTERY SIGN IN OCCLUSION OF MIDDLE CEREBRAL ARTERY - A NEGATIVE PREDICTOR FOR SPONTANEOUS RECANALISATION?

Allendoerfer J, Degner D, Merx S, von Reutern GM. Stroke Unit, Asklepios Neurologische Klinik, 63667 Bad Salzhausen, Germany.

BACKGROUND AND PURPOSE: In many studies the hyperdense middle artery sign (HMCAS) is referred to as useful sign in the diagnosis of middle cerebral artery (MCA) occlusion in acute ischemic stroke. The specificity of the HMCAS approaches 100% whereas its sensitivity is low. In some reports the HMCAS has been associated with severe neurological deficit, extensive brain damage, and poor clinical outcome. We evaluated acute stroke patients with occlusion of MCA in order to get information whether HMCAS in these patients is of predictive value in terms of early recanalisation and clinical outcome.

METHODS: In a 2 years period all patients admitted to our stroke unit within 12 hours after stroke and presenting less then 90 points in the European Stroke Scale (ESS) underwent CT scan, extracranial cw Dopplersonography (CWD) and transcranial colour-coded duplex sonography (TCCS). In case of MCA occlusion CT scan and TCCS were repeated within 24 hours. The modified Rankin Scale (mRS) was assessed on day 7 and day 30 after stroke.

RESULTS: In 31 patients we detected by Doppler Ultrasound (TCCS) an occlusion of the MCA. The HMCAS was present in 13 (42%) of our patients. There were no significant differences between patients with and without HMCAS concerning age, case fatality, mRS on day 7 and 30, and hematocrit on admission. The rate of complete recanalisation within 24 hours after admission was higher in patients without HMCAS (56%) than in those with HMCAS (10%). The rate of cardioembolic origin of stroke was higher in patients without HMCAS (72%) than in those with HMCAS (30%).

CONCLUSION: In this series MCA occlusion with HMCAS is not a marker for special poor clinical outcome in this group of severely affected patients. It seems to be that a thrombus of cardiac origin is of lower density in early CT scan and shows more often spontaneous lysis than thrombi resulting from atherosclerotic lesions.

58

PROGNOSTIC VALUE OF TRANSCRANIAL DOPPLER IN THE ACUTE PHASE OF ISCHEMIC STROKE.

C. Baracchini, R. Manara, G. Malferrari, B. Marini, M. Del Sette, G.A. Ottonello, G.P. Anzola, L. Lusiani, G.C. Landini, G. Meneghetti.

Department of Neurological Sciences, University of Padua, Italy
On behalf of the Società Interdisciplinare NeuroVascolare - S.I.N.V.

Introduction: Recent thrombolytic trials have stressed the needs to identify early markers of outcome in the acute ischemic stroke in order to improve the therapeutic approach. This study aims to verify the prognostic value of Transcranial doppler (TCD) in the acute phase of stroke.

Material and Methods: 73 patients (43 males; mean age 67.0 ± 13.4 ys) with a middle cerebral artery (MCA) ischemic stroke were categorized according to Bamford's clinical classification; all patients underwent a cerebral CT and an extra-intracranial ultrasound examination within 12 hours from clinical onset (mean 5.9±3.6 hours); CT was repeated after a week, TCD after 1 and 7 days. These data were compared with clinical course (Unified Neurological Stroke Scale: at admission, and after 7 and 14 days) and with clinical outcome (Barthel Index, BI, after 14, 30 and 90 days).

Results: In our study 52 pts were TACI, 14 PACI and 7 LACI. Cerebral CT at admission revealed early ischemic signs in 27 pts (37%). Early TCD examination disclosed an MCA occlusion in 24 patients, which recanalized in 9 cases within 7 days (6 within 24 hours); blood flow velocity asymmetry was recorded in further 30 pts; 25 patients had an internal carotid occlusion. MCA occlusion correlated with clinical TACI ($p<0.05$) but not with the presence of early signs in the CT at admission. After 3 months 32 pts (44%) were independent (BI > 60), 26 pts (35%) were dependent (BI ≤ 60). No patient with MCA occlusion was independent at 3 months. Mortality rate at 3 months was 21% (15 pts, 11 within 7 days) in the whole group, but rose to 50 % in patients with MCA occlusion and became 61% in those who did not recanalize within 24 hours.

TACI, MCA occlusion and TCD asimmetry significantly correlated ($p<0.001$, χ^2 test) both with mortality and with worse outcome (BI≤60) in survivors at 90 days.

Conclusions: TACI, MCA occlusion and TCD asimmetry are early strong predictors of poor outcome at 90 days. Moreover, TCD can identify those patients, in the TACI subgroup, who have the worst prognosis.

59

SONOGRAPHIC FEATURES OF CRANIOCERVICAL ARTERY DISSECTION

Lovrenčić-Huzjan A, Bosnar-Puretić M, Vuković V, Demarin V.
Neurology Department, University hospital “Sestre milosrdnice”, Zagreb, Vinogradska 29, fax. 385-1-376-82-82

Craniocervical artery (CCA) dissection are primary diagnosed by angiography, MR or MRA. Sonographic findings include a variety of findings, and frequently are missed due to localisation.

The aim of the study was to analyse the spectrum of sonographic findings in patients, who presented with clinical or ultrasonographic dissection of CCAs investigated in Neurology Doppler laboratory during two years period.

From January 1th 1998 to December 31th 1999. 42 patients with CCA dissection were investigated. 23 patients clinically presented with CCA dissection and in 19 ultrasonography double lumen or bifurcation stenosis with double lumen. Color and power Doppler of carotid and vertebral arteries was performed on Acuson 128XP. Color and power Doppler scans and hemodynamic spectra were analysed. The data are presented descriptively.

Out of 42 patients 4 had multivessel involvement. Out of 37 carotid dissections 6 presented with string sign, 1 string and pearl sign, 1 intimal flap, 9 double lumen, 18 bifurcation stenosis with double lumen under the plaque base, and 2 hemodynamic spectra suggesting distal occlusion. Out of 9 vertebral artery dissections 1 had intimal flap, 2 double lumens and 6 hemodynamic spectra suggesting distal occlusion. 2 subclavian arteries showed double lumen.

Color and power Doppler sonography are showing a broad spectrum of findings in CCA dissection and thus are useful methods for its screening.

60

SONOGRAPHIC MONITORING OF MIDLINE-SHIFT IN STROKE PATIENTS

E.Stolz, T. Gerriets, I. Fiss, SS Babacan, C. Algermissen, M. Kaps
Departments of Neurology Justus-Liebig University Giessen and Medical University of Lübeck, Germany

Background: Transcranial sonography (TS) enables the reliable measurement of the dislocation of the third ventricle in space occupying stroke. The aim of this study was to assess the method's ability to predict outcome in MCA stroke victims.
Methods: In 20 patients with ischaemic stroke of > 50% of the MCA territory midline shift (MLS) was monitored by TS 8 hourly within the first 48 h after symptom onset.
Results: 6 patients died due to brainstem herniation, 14 patients survived. After 16 h, the degree of MLS was significantly lower in survivors than in the patients who died.

	8 h	16 h	24 h	32 h	40 h	48 h
MLV(herniation) (SD)	**0.9 mm** (0.8)	**3.6 mm** (1.0)	**4.9 mm** (1.2)	**7.5 mm** (1.7)	**8.6 mm** (0.5)	**10.5 mm** (2.84)
MLV(survivors) (SD)	**1.1 mm** (0.7)	**1.3 mm** (0.9)	**1.7 mm** (1.1)	**1.7 mm** (1.1)	**1.7 mm** (1.2)	**2.1 mm** (1.3)
p	(0.84)	0.04	0.016	0.001	0.03	0.003

Conclusions: Sonographic measurement of MLS is able to discriminate stroke survivors from that will suffer herniation as early as 16 h after stroke onset. The method may be valuable in deciding for decompressive craniotomy.

61

Pattern of intra-and extra- cranial stenosis in Thai patients with stroke and stroke risk factors

Disya Ratanakorn,M.D., Charungthai Dejthevaporn,M.D.
Division of Neurology, Department of Medicine
Faculty of Medicine, Ramathibodi Hospital
Mahidol University, Bangkok, Thailand

Although ischemic cerebrovascular disease (CVD) forms 70% of all stroke in Thailand where the prevalence of stroke was reported as 6.9 / 1000 population, extracranial carotid artery stenosis (ECAS) was believed to be relatively rare. The angiographic study of 129 patients with acute stroke showed ECAS in only 5%, which was relatively low compared to 17% in British patients reported in the early 1960's. In 1994, a study using carotid duplex in acute stroke patients showed an amazingly high prevalence of ECAS with 56% due to inadequate technique and criteria. We studied 100 consecutive patients referred to our Neurosonology Laboratory during May to October 1998 with carotid duplex and transcranial Doppler ultrasonography. Using modified TOAST criteria, 70 patients had CVD (gr1), 30 patients had associated stroke risk factors without CVD (gr2). The mean age was 59.8+/-13.8 yr in gr1, 61.2+/-13.7 yr in gr2, and the ratio of male:female was 1:1.3 in gr1, and 1:1 in gr2 . In gr1: there were 17.4% of EICAS , 64.8% of ICS, and 9.3% of tandem lesions. In gr 2: There were 13.3% of EICAS , 38.1% of ICS , and 14.3% of tandem lesions. Multivariate analysis of risk factors including age, sex, diabetes mellitus, hypertension, hyperlipidemia, smoking, pills did not show significant association between these risk factors and EICAS, ICS, and tandem lesions.

In conclusion, ICS is still the major finding in stroke patients and asymptomatic patients with stroke risk factors. However, the finding of ECAS in stroke seems to be higher compared to that of 30 years ago (17.4% vs 5%) in spite of different investigation techniques. There is also a high percentage (13.3%) of ECAS in the patients without stroke. Therefore, detection of ECAS in acute stroke Thai patients is warranted, as well as in asymptomatic patients with stroke risk factors, since carotid endarterectomy has been proved to be effective in both groups of patients, as well as in those who have tandem lesions.

62

Longitudinal Follow-up of intracranial arterial stenosis with Transcranial Doppler Ultrasonography

Sun U. Kown, M.D., Jae H. Lee, M.D., Jong S. Kim, M.D.
Department of Neurology, Asan Medical Center, University of Ulsan, Seoul, Korea

Background and Purpose : The natural history of intracranial arterial stenoses remains unknown. To investigate prognosis of the stenoses in the intracranial cerebral arteries and the possible role of clinical prognostic factors, we conducted a prospective study using transcranial Doppler (TCD) ultrasonography. ***Methods*** : We performed TCD study on 82 stroke patients with angiographically documented stenosis of middle cerebral artery (MCA) or basilar artery (BA). The findings were compared to repeat TCD studies conducted more than 2 months apart with respect to changes in mean flow velocities (mFV) of the stenotic segment. We analyzed the clinical data of all patients including risk factors of atherosclerosis, electrocardiogram, echocardiogram, and patterns of stenosis, which may affect the natural history of arterial stenosis. ***Results*** : Ninety seven arteries (47 left MCA, 31 right MCA, and 19 BA) from 82 patients (64 men and 18 women; mean age 56.6 years) were serially examined. During a mean follow-up period of 12.0 months, 23 (23.7%) arteries had TCD evidence of stenosis progression and 25 (25.8%) showed stenosis regression on TCD. BAs had better prognosis than MCAs ($p<0.05$), and arteries with symptomatic stenosis had better than arteries with asymptomatic ($p<0.05$). Age, sex, degree of stenosis, presence of source of cardioembolism, or any risk factors of atherosclerosis were not associated with the prognosis of the stenosis. ***Conclusion*** : These findings suggest that stenoses of intracranial arteries are dynamic lesions, and that they can evolve or regress after relatively short periods. There are no reliable predictive factors of the natural course except for symptomatic stenosis and BA involvement. TCD can noninvasively detect these changes over time.

63

THROMBOLYTIC EFFECTS OF 1 MHZ STANDARD DIAGNOSTIC ULTRASOUND

K. SPENGOS, S. BEHRENS, M. DAFFERTSHOFER, C.E. DEMPFLE, M. HENNERICI

Dept. of Neurology, Universitätsklinikum Mannheim, University of Heidelberg, Germany

Neurological outcome in acute stroke from MCA occlusion depends on the time until vessel recanalization. Thrombolysis with rt-PA within a short time window after stroke onset is an efficient therapy. Non-thermal effects of low-frequency ultrasound (US) have been shown to accelerate enzymatic drug mediated fibrinolysis in vitro. We examined the effects of a commercially available standard 1MHz pulsed-wave probe on rt-PA-mediated thrombolysis in a flow model in vitro.
Pure fibrin clots were placed in a continuous pressure flow model and all treated with rt-PA. Transtemporal application through a postmortem skull or direct insonation (1 MHz; SPTA: 0,5 W/cm^2; pulse repitition frequency: 16 kHz, sample volume: 25mm; Multidop X4, DWL, Sipplingen, Germany) significantly ($p<0,001$) shortened recanalization time (21,1 and 20,8 vs. 34,4 min), increased perfusion flow (2,03 and 2,23 vs. 0,45 ml/min) and reperfusion fluid weight (60,9 and 67 vs. 13,4 g) compared with rt-PA mediated thrombolysis only. Recanalization rate was 90-100% in the rt-PA/US groups vs. 30% in the rt-PA group within the exposure period of 30 min.
Our results show efficacy of low intnsity 1 MHz US, even when applied through the temporal bone, in accelerating rt-PA mediated thrombolysis in vitro and are in accordance with several other studies examining thrombolysis in perpheral or coronary vessels. This new aspect makes further experimental studies necessary, in order to examine potential use of transcranial applied US as an accelerator of acute thrombolytic stroke therapy.

64

ENHANCEMENT OF IN-VITRO-THROMBOLYSIS BY LOW-FREQUENCY ULTRASOUND

Nedelmann M, BM Eicke, A Heimann, O Kempski, E Liercke, HC Hopf

University Hospital of Mainz, Department of Neurology, Germany

Acceleration of clot lysis to restore circulation may limit the extent of brain injury and improve clinical outcome after stroke. The use of thrombolytic agents in acute ischaemic infarction, however, only showed modest benefit in clinical trials.
Potentially, low-frequency ultrasound may enhance the effect of thrombolytic agents. The purpose of our study was to assess the efficacy of low-frequency ultrasound alone and in combination with rt-PA for its potential to accelerate in-vitro-thrombolysis.
In-vitro-thrombolysis of fresh human blood clots with and without rt-PA (3μg/ml) was studied by using 20 kHz cw-ultrasound (KLN, Germany) at power levels of 0.15, 0.35 and 0.5 W/cm² at different exposure times (5, 10 and 20 min). The age of the investigated thrombi in each group ranged from 3 to 5 hours. Loss in weight of each blood clot was used to measure the extent of thrombolysis. The number of treated thrombi in each group was 10. Experiments were carried out in phosphate-buffered saline, at a temperature of 37°C, in an open-loop flow system with a flow rate of 15 ml/min.
The use of ultrasound alone showed a significant thrombolytic effect in each studied power level and exposure time (weight loss ranging from 33,2% at 0,35 W/cm² and 5 min to 60,7% at 0,5 W/cm² and 10 min), as compared to a control group (24,2%). There was a significant correlation between the extent of weight loss and the increase in power and exposure time. The combination of ultrasound (0.35 W/cm², 10 min) and rt-PA significantly enhanced thrombolysis (65,2%) compared to rt-PA alone (48,4%). Lysis was more effective in fresh thrombi. At studied power levels and exposure times, there was no measurable rise in temperature of the medium, even when circulation of the medium was stopped.
These data suggest that use of low-frequency ultrasound has the potential to increase the efficacy of thrombolysis and therefore may be a promising tool to develop an alternative or addition to current treatment modalities of acute stroke.

Abstracts of Posters

65

MICROEMBOLIC SIGNAL DESCRIPTION - A REAPPRAISAL BASED ON A CUSTOMIZED DIGITAL POST-PROCESSING SYSTEM

W.H. Mess, J.M. Willigers, L.A.F. Ledoux, A.P.G. Hoeks

CARIM, Maastricht University, The Netherlands

The high variability in presence and signature of microembolic signals (MES) detected with TCD in the middle cerebral artery (MCA) can not be explained with the currently available published data.
We applied customized post-processing on the radio frequency (RF) signal of a standard TCD system (DWL Multidop X 4), which was sampled on an external PC at 16 MHz. The spatial resolution was better than 2 mm, depending only on the length of the ultrasound burst emitted. The amplitude of clutter-filtered RF signals was color-coded and plotted as a function of time and depth (range 30 mm). Additionally, 128 point FFTs (50% temporal overlap) were calculated, visualizing conventionally both the background Doppler spectrum and the MES.
We evaluated 120 MES from two patients during cardiac surgery, which in both patients showed comparable properties. The MES appeared in the RF amplitude plot as straight lines of increased intensity, indicating that the velocity did not change while passing through the ultrasound beam. The velocity calculated from the amplitude plot never exceeded the background Doppler spectrum and tended to be slower than been derived from FFT. Various "MES patterns" could be identified with respect to the depth range at which the MES were visible. Many MES changed their direction at a specific depth, suggesting that the MES entered an M2 artery or the anterior cerebral artery. With FFT analysis these MES were present in both the positive and negative frequency spectrum.
It is concluded that the previously reported variability of MES is an artefact caused by the relatively large amplitudes and depth ranges, that is sample volumes, considered.

66

DOPPLER SIGNAL AMPLITUDE CHANGES DURING CARDIAC SURGERY

W.H. Mess, L.A. Walda, A.P.G. Hoeks

CARIM, Maastricht University, The Netherlands

Waterbath studies suggest that the amplitude of the Doppler signal backscattered from a sample volume in a blood vessel may increase up to four times when the hematocrit decreases from physiological values to 15-20%. Significant hematocrit changes occur during cardiac surgery due to the delutional effect of extracorporal circulation (EC). Since the calculation of microembolic signal (MES) intensity includes a comparison with the background signal, large Doppler amplitude changes could have a serious impact on the differentiation between particulate and gaseous MES.
We measured in two patients before and after the introduction of EC the Doppler signal from the middle cerebral artery (MCA) with a standard TCD machine (DWL X 4). The Doppler audio signal was recorded on DAT tape and its instantaneous amplitude was afterwards detected with a wideband RMS multimeter and processed by specially designed software. An increase of 35% (684mV ± 43[SD] vs. 505mV ± 37[SD]) and 17% (848mV±10[SD] vs. 724mV ± 11[SD]) was measured. With the initiation of EC a transient Doppler amplitude peak was noticed (842mv; 67% increase vs pre EC and 974mV; 35% resp.). The hematocrit values were 32 vs 16 and 36 vs 23, respectively.
We demonstrated in vivo that after the initiation of EC, and hence a marked decrease of the hematocrit, the Doppler amplitude of the MCA signal only showed a modest increase, which is neglegible for the calculation of MES intensities. Possibly, a lowered fibrinogen (52% decrease and 45% resp.), which is also a consequence of the dilution, partially outweighs the effect of the lowered hematocrit on the Doppler amplitude as seen with waterbath analysis.

67

DIAGNOSIS OF INTRACARDIAC R-L SHUNT WITH TRANSCRANIAL COLOR FLOW IMAGING USING ONE-DROP-METHOD OF HORIZON[R]

T Terasaki, S Orita, M Shimamura, Y Hashimoto and M Uchino

Department of Strokology and Neurology, Kumamoto City Hospital, Kumamoto, Japan
Department of Neurology, Kumamoto University School of Medicine, Kumamoto, Japan

Aim: To clarify the usefulness of one-drop-method (ODM) of Horizon[R] (diazepam solution for injection, Yamanouchi co. Japan) in terms of detecting high intensity transient signals (HITS) that implies intracardiac right to left shunt (R-L shunt) with transcranial color flow imaging (TC-CFI).
Subject: 27 cases were studied with transesophageal echocardiography to investigate the presence of R-L shunt. 30 vessels (middle cerebral artery 19, basilar artery 11) of 16 cases (male 11, female 5, age 56.5 years old) with R-L shunt and 15 vessels (middle cerebral artery 12, basilar artery 3) of 11 cases (male 9, female 2, age 58.6years old) without R-L shunt were studied.
Methods: Agitated cold saline (9 ml with 1 ml air) was injected from the cubital vein. Intracranial doppler flow signal was monitored by TC-CFI (Ultramark 9, ATL) to detect HITS for 30 seconds after injection under Valsalva maneuver. Another 30 seconds of monitoring was performed after the injection of agitated cold saline with one drop (approximately 0.05 ml) of Horizon[R] mixed from the 3-way connector (one-drop-method). We investigated the influence of ODM on the frequency and the number of detected HITS.
Result: Among the cases having R-L shunt, HITS were detected in 10 vessels (33.3%) of 7 cases (43.8%) without ODM, and 16 vessels (53.3%) of 10 cases (62.5%) with ODM. The number of HITS increased in 13 vessels (43.3%) of 7 cases (43.8%). On the other hand, no HITS were detected regardless of ODM among the patients without R-L shunt.
Conclusion: ODM is a useful method to increase the detectability of HITS in patients with R-L shunt using TC-CFI.

68

MICROEMBOLIC SIGNAL ANALYSIS BASED ON A DIGITAL RADIOFREQUENCY SYSTEM.

J.M. Willigers, W.H. Mess, L.A.F. Ledoux, A.P.G. Hoeks
CARIM, Maastricht University, The Netherlands

To allow for customized post processing of micro embolic signals (MES) the radio frequency (RF) signal of a standard TCD system (DWL Multidop X4) is digitized and stored on hard disk. From the TCD system the RF-signal, the emission trigger and the synchronous sample clock are made externally available and are connected to a custom-made PC-data acquisition interface. This interface digitizes the RF-signals, stores them into the PC-memory, where after they are transferred to hard disk. A single recording of RF-signals can cover a depth range of 30 mm lasting for 10 seconds, for a sample frequency of 16 MHz, a pulse repetition frequency of 6 kHz and 64 MB PC-memory.
The actual spatial resolution of the acquired RF-signals is not limited by the acquisition and is only dependent on the length of the ultrasound burst transmitted. In practice, the spatial resolution is better than 2 mm. MES can be acquired by pressing a switch when an emboli is acoustically noticed. The RF-signals within one second before and one second after pressing the switch are transferred to the hard disk. From these RF-signals, Doppler spectra can be determined. The number, length, position and inter spacing of the receiver gates can be chosen freely at post-processing. Also the amplitude of the MES as function of time and depth can be visualized. Since all the spatial information is retained, the MES characteristics in terms of amplitude and velocity can be evaluated in time and along the insonated vessel.
The system offers the opportunity to enhance the knowledge about temporal and spatial MES characteristics and may contribute to automated detection of MES.

69

EMBOLIC SIGNAL VARIATION IN PATIENTS WITH ASYMPTOMATIC CAROTID ARTERY STENOSIS.

A Abbott (nee Harris), B Chambers, J Stork, C Levi, C Bladin, G Donnan.
National Stroke Research Institute, Austin and Repatriation Medical Centre, Victoria and the Neurology Department, John Hunter Hospital, NSW, 2305.

It is not known how results of embolic signal (ES) detection vary over time in patients with asymptomatic carotid stenosis. Such information is necessary in planning studies to see if this technique can be used to predict stroke symptoms in such patients. The aim was to test the variability over time of Transcranial Doppler ES detection in patients with asymptomatic carotid stenosis. 160 arteries from 146 asymptomatic patients with 60-99% carotid stenosis had a baseline one hour embolus detection study. A further one-hour study was done the same day or up to 30 months apart from this study. The off-line six-decibel threshold microemboli positivity and negativity results for the paired studies were compared. 456 repeat arterial studies were performed the same day or within 30 months of the initial study. Differing results of ES detection were seen in 7% of 113 studies performed the same day, 11% of 56 studies 1-14 days apart, 12% of 57 studies 15 days to less than 6 months apart and 15% of 97 studies 6-11 months apart. For 133 studies performed 12 to 30 months apart from an initial study, differing results were seen in 9 to 16% of cases. Variability in ES detection appears to increase with time. This implies that the carotid disease process is a dynamic one. ES detection should be repeated serially to evaluate the value of this technique in predicting stroke symptoms.

70

INHIBITION OF TIA AND CEREBRAL MICROEMBOLI BY ACETYLSALICYLIC ACID IN ESSENTIAL THROMBOCYTHEMIA

T. Blaser, S. Krueger, R. Kross, G. Lutze*, M. Goertler
Department of Neurology, *Insitute of Clinical Chemistry
Otto-von-Guericke University Magdeburg, Germany

Background: Up to 60% of patients with essential thrombocythemia present neurological symptoms. Platelet thrombi in the arterial microvasculature induced by thrombocytosis and platelet hyperaggregability are considered the underlying pathology.
Patient and Methods: We present a 69-year-old man with recurrent bilateral TIAs which completely recovered after 10 to 30 minutes. Cranial CT was normal. Diagnostic work up revealed no cardiac or arterial findings associated with an increased risk of embolism. Medical history showed a moderate hypertension and a long lasting nicotine abuse. Embolus detection found 18 microemboli/hour in both middle cerebral arteries. Venous blood samples revealed thrombocytosis (682 x 10^9/L) with circulating platelet aggregates and mega-platelets. Bone marrow biopsy confirmed the diagnosis of essential thrombocythemia.
Results: Acetylsalicylic acid, initiated by an intravenous bolus of 500 mg and continued orally with 300 mg/day, abolished further ischemic events as well as transcranial Doppler detected microemboli. This corresponded with inhibited platelet aggregability in aggregation tests. Ischemic events and microemboli reappeared after treatment interruption. Recommencement of therapy stopped both symptoms and microemboli corresponding to reestablished inhibition in platelet aggregation tests.
Conclusions: Our findings suggest, that microemboli detected in this patient corresponded to circulating platelet aggregates which were suppressed by acetylsalicylic acid and were responsible for cerebral ischemia.

71

EFFECT OF ANTITHROMBOTIC AGENTS ON CEREBRAL MICROEMBOLI IN PATIENTS WITH SYMPTOMATIC ARTERIAL STENOSIS

M. Goertler, T. Blaser, S. Krueger, C.-W. Wallesch, G. Lutze*
Department of Neurology, *Insitute of Clinical Chemistry
Otto-von-Guericke University Magdeburg, Germany

Background: Antithrombotic agents, i.e. anticoagulants and antiplatelet drugs, are considered the therapy of choice after an ischemic event due to symptomatic arterial stenosis. Reduction of cerebral embolism is the presumed mechanism.
Patients and Methods: Thirty patients (24 men, mean age 60.0+/-13 years) with symptomatic arterial stenosis and clinical symptoms within the last 30 days underwent recurrent one-hour bilateral embolus detection before and after initiation of an antithrombotic prevention. Based on clinical decisions, 15 patients received antiplatelet agents, i.e. acetylsalicylic acid, ticlopidine or clopidogrel, whereas 15 were set on intravenous heparin (aPTT 2-fold of baseline). Patients in both groups did not differ by their main clinical characteristics and diagnostic findings.
Results: 20.0 microemboli/hour (mean; range 0-59) were detected in patients before antiplatelet medication compared to 18.0 (1-54) before heparin (n.s.). In patients on antiplatelet drugs mean number of microemboli decreased to 0.3 (range, 0-3) (P=0.001), whereas their number was unchanged in those receiving heparin (mean/hour, 17.1; range, 2-57). After anticoagulation was switched to an antiplatelet therapy in 11 of the 15 patients, microemboli decreased to 0.1 (mean/hour; range, 0-1) (P=0.003).
Conclusions: Antiplatelet agents but not an anticoagulation with intravenous heparin reduce transcranial Doppler detected microemboli originating from symptomatic arterial stenoses.

72

DETECTION OF CEREBRAL MICROEMBOLI IN PROSTHETIC HEART VALVE PATIENTS

A.Kuznetsov, A.Lupeev, Yu.Kolbin, M.Odinak, Yu.Shevchenko, I.Voznyuk
Military Medical Academy, St.-Petersburg, Russia

The transcranial Doppler sonography allows to register microembolus passage through the cerebral vessels. The purpose of this study was to evaluate the incidence and frequency of the microembolic signals (MES) in patients with prosthetic heart valves (PHV), and also to determine its contributing factors and clinical importance.
We studied 15 patients with mechanical PHV in mitral (8 patients) or aortal (7 patients) position 4 to 16 years after heart surgery. We carried out 30-minute transcranial Doppler monitoring of the middle cerebral artery with calculation of the number and intensity of MES in an on-line and off-line mode with the observer on the device «Sonomed-300» («Spectromed», Moscow, Russia).
MES are found out in 3 of 15 patients (20%). The number of MES per 30 minutes was 3, 4, and 7, accordingly. Relative MES intensity increase was less than 30 dB, that testified to their material nature. MES are found out in two patients with PHV dysfunction and in one patient with recent ischemic stroke. MES are not found out in the patients with normal function of PHV. There was no correlation between the MES number and PHV position, and the MES number and intensity of anticoagulant therapy.
Thus, the cerebral microembolism in PHV is often event. Their occurrence is connected to PHV dysfunction and associated with cerebral ischemic events.

73

ASSESSMENT OF MES DURING CAROTID ENDOVASCULAR PROCEDURES

O Martinelli, ***B Gossetti, R Stumpo, A Siani, F Tommasini*, F Benedetti-Valentini***
2nd Chair of Vascular Surgery and *Anesthesiology Department of "La Sapienza" University of Rome (Italy)

The benefits of carotid endarterectomy (CEA) has been validated by several multicenter trials while the value of carotid artery stenting is still controversial because of the risk of intraprocedural cerebral embolism.
Purpose: to evaluate the usefulness of transcranial Doppler (TCD) periprocedural monitoring during percutaneous angioplasty (PTA) and stenting of the supraortic vessels.
Methods: over a 12 months period, 4 patients underwent PTA + stenting for internal carotid artery (ICA) recurrent stenosis following CEA, 1 for severe stenosis of the left common carotid artery 3 cm above its origin and 1 for a severe innominate artery stenosis. The percutaneous technique included standard retrograde femoral artery access with ballooon dilatation and stent deployement in all cases. No intraluminal protection was used. Before treatment, all patients were submitted to 30' TCD monitoring in order to detect microembolic signals (MES) which were recorded only in 1 case. Intraprocedurally, TCD monitoring was performed in order to evaluate cerebral blood flow and evidence of MES from the beginning to the end of endovascular treatment.
Results: preoperative TCD monitoring showed isolated MES in 1 patient with recurrent ICA stenosis. During endovascular procedure the highest incidence of MES were recorded during catheter introduction into the operated artery and retraction in all cases. MES were also detected during stent deployement. MES were asymptomatic in all patients but 1 with innominate artery disease who had a shower of MES during stenting followed by a minor stroke which remitted completely within 7 days. A decrease of mean blood flow velocity in ipsilateral middle cerebral artery was always recorded during balloon inflation In one case that decrease was critical but so short to be at no risk of ischemia.
Conclusion: TCD monitoring allows to identify, preprocedurally, the lesions at high-risk for microembolic complications. During percutaneous treatment of supraortic vessels, the evidence of > 10/min MES should suggest the need of intraluminal cerebral protection.

74

TRANSCRANIAL DOPPLER DETECTION OF MICROEMBOLI IN CHINESE PATIENTS WITH ACUTE ISCHEMIC STROKE

Ni X.S., Zhu W. H. Wang C., Department of Neurology, Drum Tower Hospital, Nanjing University Medical College, Nanjing 210008, P.R. China

Objectives: Transcranial Doppler(TCD) detection of cerebral arterial microemboli signal(MES) were performed in Chinese patients with acute ischemic stroke to investigate the incidence and its clinical significance. **Methods:** We prospectively studied 115 Chinese patients with acute ischemic stroke of anterior circulation. 53 patients had potential source of emboli, including cardiogenic embolism (n=29), middle cerebral artery(MCA) stenosis(n=16) and carotid stenosis (n=8). All patients were performed bilateral MCA TCD monitoring for 30–60 (41.98±9.03)min using 2 MHz bigated probes within 5h–7d(3.39±1.52d) after onset of symptoms. **Results:** MES were detected in 4.34%(5/115) patients. MES were more frequent in cardiogenic embolism (3/29), MCA stenosis (2/16) than in carotid stenosis(0/8). **Conclusions:** The incidence of MES in Chinese patients with acute ischemic stroke was significantly lower than that in west countries. The main sources of MES in Chinese patients with acute ischemic stroke were the cardiogenic embolism and intracranial arterial stenosis, not the carotid stenosis.

75

THE CARDIOEMBOLIC SOURCES OF SMALL RISK FOR ISCHEMIC BRAIN DISEASE

Dragan Tavciovski, Ranko Raicevic*, Aco Jovicic*, Momcilo Krgovic, Dragana Djordjevic*, Toplica Lepic*, Bratislav Magdic*.Department of Cardiology,Department of Neurology*,Military Medical Academy,Belgrade ,FR Yugoslavia

Introduction.
Ischemic brain disease (IBD) represents unique clinical entity with various ethiological factors. Embolic mechanisms of development with thrombotic material of cardiac origin is the cause in 20-50% of the cases.The aim of the study was to determine the significance and sensitivity of TEE in detection of cardiac abnormalities which are considered to be the small risc source in patients with IBD in which the embolic mechanism of disease development was suspected.
Methods and results.
We examined 60 patients with acute acute IBD, proved according to clinical and radiological criteria, of probably cardioembolic development mechanism and by transthoracal(TTE) and TEE peformed by two examiners in order to exclude bias.Significance of diferences in detection of cardiac abnormalities was determined by statistical calculations.
In patients group examined by TEE mitral valve prolaps was detected in 19 patients (was detected in 14 cases when TTE was used). Atrial septal aneurism was detected in 8 patients by TEE and with only 2 positive finding when TTE was used. Spontaneous echo contrast was seen in 6 cases only by TEE method.
Conclusions.
According to our results,we can conclude that TEE is significantly more sensitive diagnostic method for detection of small risk cardioembolic sources in development of IBD which is specially related to younger patients.

76

DETECTION OF EMBOLIC SIGNALS IN ASYMPTOMATIC SUBJECTS WITH NON-VALVULAR ATRIAL FIBRILLATION; THE EFFECTS OF ANTICOAGULATION

K Tinkler, M Cullinane, Z Kaposzta, HS Markus.

Royal Free Hospital, King's College Hospital & St. George's Hospital Medical School, London, UK.

Introduction: Non-Valvular atrial fibrillation (NVAF) has an annual stroke risk of approximately 5%. Current treatment includes anticoagulation to reduce the risk of cardiac embolism. Transcranial Doppler (TCD) may be used to screen for embolic signals (ES) in this group and to monitor the effects of anticoagulation.

Methods: 183 asymptomatic subjects were investigated. 21 did not have an acoustic window. The resulting groups comprised of 1- taking warfarin (n=70) mean(SD) age 71.6(6.5)yrs, 2- not taking warfarin (n=62) mean(SD) age 74.7(9.1)yrs and 3- a control group (n=30) mean(SD) age 71.9(7.9)yrs in sinus rhythm. TCD recordings were performed on two occasions from bilateral middle cerebral arteries for 1 hour. All data was recorded on to DAT for blinded analysis.

Results: Following the first recording ES were detected in both the NVAF groups but not in the controls: non-warfarin(4) patients vs controls(0) patients p=0.16. Warfarin(2) vs controls(0) p=0.35. After repeating the TCD recording in both the NVAF groups the number of ES positive non-warfarin subjects(7) was significantly higher than the ES positive warfarin subjects(2), p=0.045. The mean(SD) number of ES detected in the non-warfarin group was also higher than the warfarin group; 0.19(0.57) vs 0.03(0.17) p=0.04 (Mann-Whitney U). Marked variability in ES detection was seen by repeating the TCD recording, the number of ES positive subjects doubled in the non-warfarin group.

Conclusion: ES are infrequent in all patients with NVAF but more common in subjects not taking warfarin. Marked temporal variability was seen.

77

CORRELATIONS OF CEREBRAL MICROEMBOLY IN PATIENTS WITH CAROTID ATHEROSCLEROSIS

TOMILIN A. A., MD; LAGODA O. V. MD; DJIBLADZE D.N., MD, PH.D.

Institute of Neurology, Moscow, Russia

Background and purpose. The importance of TCD as a method of detection cerebral microemboly is well known. Though, the significance of detected microembolic signals isn't obvious. The majority of spontaneous microembolic signals doesn't cause the development of neurological symptoms.

Materials and Methods. We examined 96 arteries of 60 patients with atherosclerotic carotid stenoses. There were two groups of patients: with symptomatic and "silence" carotid stenoses. We studied characteristics of cerebral microemboly according to the symptoms, severity of carotid stenoses, morphology of plaques, and fibrinogen level. TCD of cerebral blood flow in middle cerebral arteries was detected using "Pioneer TC2020" system ("Pioneer", USA).

Results. Frequency of cerebral microemboly in the group of patients with symptomatic carotid stenoses was significantly higher (31% vs. 14%). We found a trend to higher frequency of microembolic signals in cases of high-grade carotid stenoses. Microembolic signals were detected in 4% in the group of patients with small carotid stenoses, in 22% in the group of patients with moderate carotid stenoses. In the groups of patients with high-grade and subtotal carotid stenoses frequency of microembolic signals was 37.5% and 43% respectively. Frequency of cerebral microemboly depended on plaque morphology and was higher in cases of unstable plaques. When the plaque was fibrous we didn't detect any microembolic signals. Frequency of microembolic signals in cases of hypodence plaques was about 40%. In cases of intraplaque hemorrhage or plaque's ulceration microembolic signals were observed in 75%. Comparing the results in the group of patients with ulcerated plaques or intraplaque hemorrhages with other groups, we found higher frequency in the first group (72% and 14% respectively).

Conclusions. Our results of higher frequency of microembolic signals in patients with carotid atherosclerosis are in agreement with the results of other authors. But it's clear that not all microembolic episodes are clinically significant. The genesis of development of embolism has a straight line a correlation with a morphology of atherosclerotic plaques and can be realised at a different degree of a carotid stenósis. The cerebral microembolism correlates with the unstable and ulcerated atherosclerotic plaques.

78

THE DIAGNOSTIC VALUE OF TRANSCRANIAL DOPPLER ULTRASONOGRAPHY IN PATIENTS WITH A RECENT TIA OR MINOR STROKE: POTENTIAL CARDIAC SOURCE OF EMBOLISM. A SYSTEMATIC REVIEW.

Annemarie D Wijnhoud, Peter J Koudstaal, Diederik WJ Dippel
Department of Neurology, University Hospital Rotterdam, the Netherlands

Background: Several studies suggest that in stroke patients with a potential cardiac source of embolism (PCSE) High Intensity Transient Signals (HITS) are not uncommon. However, these studies have yielded widely different results and the diagnostic value of TCD in distinguishing between the presence or absence of a PCSE in stroke patients is not established.

Methods: We searched NLM Medline for published studies on TCD in stroke or TIA patients. These studies had to meet the following criteria: comparison with an independent gold standard, absence of workup bias and review bias. PCSE should have been defined according to the TOAST criteria or an analogous method of classification. Patients with a carotid artery stenosis were excluded. Of each study we computed the sensitivity and specificity for PCSE. The data were then combined in a summary ROC curve. This curve was estimated by logit transformation of sensitivity and 1-specificity and after that, by fitting the data using linear regression, as suggested by Moses et al, Stat Med. 1993;12:1293-316.

Results: Seven studies met our criteria. The major difference between the studies was the level of the intensity threshold for identification of HITS. Four studies used an intensity threshold of 7 dB or higher (dots, continuous line), Three studies used an intensity threshold of 3 or 4 dB (asterisques, dashed line). The dotted line in the figure indicates the upper limit of the predefined range of interest, no data are available beyond that line.

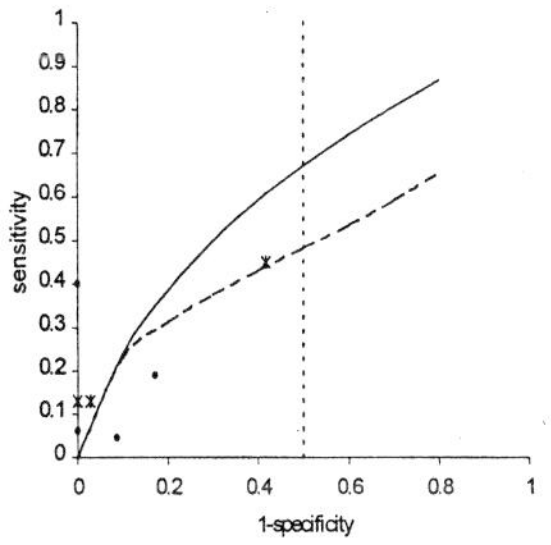

Conclusion: Our analysis suggests that for the purpose of distinguishing between patients with and patients without a PCSE, an intensity threshold for HITS detection by TCD of at least 7 dB may be optimal. Whether a further distinction between low and high risk cardiac sources of embolism would improve the summary ROC curve remains to be studied.

79

MIDDLE CEREBRAL ARTERY FLOW PARAMETERS IN PATIENTS WITH INTERNAL CAROTID REDUDANCY

A.Berchio, E.Rolfo, R.Mingozzi, C.Valenzano
D.E.A. Osservazione Medicina - A.S.O. San Giovanni Battista Torino (Italy)

The role of the redundant internal carotid artery (kinks, coils and loops)as stroke risk factor is still controversial. The aim of the paper is to relate the middle cerebral artery (MCA) flow paramters recorded in M1 with the ones recorded in omolateral internal carotid artery (ICA) with extra-cranial redudancy.

SUBJECTS AND METHODS

In the last term of 1999 an eco-colour doppler was given to 180 external pazients. Among these subjects, 27 bringers of ICA were detected with redudancies (7 of them with bilateral redudancies).In these patients the following was examined: •peak systolic velocity •end diastolic velocity •some derived parameters: 1)mean flow velocity 2)P.I.(Gosling pulsatility index) 3) R.I.(Pourcelot resistence index).ECST method > 30° ICA stenosis bringers were excluded. Pazients with > 50% MCA stenosis were also excluded.

RESULTS

Average age in redudancies bringers was 67,9 ± 14,9. 34 carotids were examined. Hypertension, the most frequent risk factor for atherosclerosis, was present in 70% of subjects. As regard the ICA values, MCA varations in the velocities were noticed: (systolic, diastolic, mean) although they did not reach any significative statistics. Statistacally relevant values were observed between the ICA and MCA P.I. and R.I. , respectively: p< 0,005 for P.I. and p< 0,0006 for the R.I.

DISCUSSION

The frequency of carotid redudancy, quite high among the people examined, is indeed to be correlated to a rather high average age and the concomitance of hypertension. The reduction of arterial vascular resistence might be due to the activation of a compensatory mechanism to flow reduction due to ICA tortuosity. Therefore, these patients might be considered at risk because of a vascular disease on a haemodynamic basis.

80

ULTRASOUND OF THE SUPERIOR OPHTHALMIC VEIN (SOV) - A NEW METHOD FOR NEUROLOGISTS?

JG Heckmann, A Bickel, S Leis, MJ Hilz, H Erxleben, B Neundörfer, Deptartment of Neurology, University of Erlangen-Nuremberg, Germany

Background and Purpose: In a pilot study, colour Doppler flow imaging (CDFI) of the superior ophthalmic vein (SOV) appeared to detect intracranial *hypo*tension due to an enlargement of the SOV (Lancet 1999;354:826). In contrast to this, enlargement of the SOV was found by CCT (J Neurosurg 1997;86:893) in association with intracranial *hyper*tension. To evaluate whether CDFI of the SOV can be used in clinical neurology and to present normal values correlating to intracranial pressure.

Methods: The study included 21 orbita CDFI investigations (Acuson 128 XP, Mountain View, CA, USA; 7 Mhz linear scan transducer, low-transmission-output power setting <50mW/cm^2, depth 50 mm) of 4 healthy volunteers and 8 non-cerebral diseased patients(7f,5m; mean age 41.5$\pm$14 y). In 8 patients lumbar puncture was performed and data on the CSF-opening pressure were available. The diameter of the SOV was evaluated using CDFI, as was the maximum flow velocity. In addition the time of the complete ultrasound examination was measured.

Results: In all subjects at least one SOV was clearly detected and could be analysed. In 3 subjects the right orbita was not investigated due to unclear anatomical situations. The normal diameter values of the SOV are 2.3$\pm$0.4mm (left) and 2.4$\pm$0.3mm (right). The correlation within the normal ranges is poor (p>0.05;CSF-pressure 12.1$\pm$1.2cm H_2O). In all measurements the maximum venous blood flow velocity was below 10 cm/sec. All CDFI-invetigations were perfomed in less than 20 minutes.

Conclusions: CDFI of the SOV is an easy and quick examination. It provides useful information about the venous status of the orbit. The extent to which the diameter of the SOV correlates with changed intracranial pressure needs further evaluation.

81

ULTRASOUND DIAGNOSTIC AND DETERMINATIONT OF SURGICAL TACTICS ON MULTIPLE ATHEROSKLEROSIS

T.V.Kaminskaia[1], M.D., A.V. Tolkachev[1], M.D, V.A.Yanushko[2], M.D.
[1] Diagnostic Centre, Minsk, Republic of Belarus
[2] Republic cardio-vascular Centre, Minsk, Republic of Belarus

Purpose: There is the impotent especiales of the occlusiv atherosclerotic process such as plural forms of clinical manifestations, a different temps of its development and the involvement a some regions of vessels. It is known that similar combination is significantly make worse the results of surgical correction in one of bassins and is increase the ischemic complications in the other injuried vessels zone. The purpose of this investigation was to study the spreading of the combined atherosclerotic injuries of major arteries of lower extremities (MALE) and brachio-cephalic arteries (BCA) of patients with obliterating Atherosclerosis(OA) of lower extremities, determination of the efficiency of Doppler spectrum analysis(DSA) in the diagnosis this combined vascular pathology.

Subjects and Methods: 213 patients(198 men,15 women,mean age 60 years) with OA of lower extremities have been examened with the use of clinical-Doppler method: DSA peripheral vessels and BCA sone.

Results: It have been determined that injuries of MALE on the aortae-iliac levels(syndrome Lerische) and multilevel obliterations of the peripheral vessels are combined with OA brachio- cephalic arteries in 70,4% of the cases. They have isolated character in 47% and involving carotid arteries primarely. They are multiplyed in 53% of the cases and "carotid + vertebral" arteries type occurs more often. The method of DSA was verified by R-angiography. The diagnostic accurancy with stenosis of 50-75% lumen of vessels is 94,6% and with severe stenosis or occlusions is 100%.

Summary: So, the significant spreading of the combined atherosclerotic injuries of MALE and BCA of patients with OA of lower extremities has been determined. The high diagnostic accuracy of noninvasive ultrasound method of DSA in combined vascular pathology diagnosis has been defined. This makes easy essentially the determination of the optimal curative tactic and the stages of surgical treatment of atherosclerosis, namely, step operations or step-by-step operations.

82

CEREBRAL HEMODYNAMICS DURING VENTRICULAR FIBRILLATION

C. Lund, E. Fosse*, R. Brucher, D. Russell. Depts of Neurology and Thoracic surgery*, The National Hospital, Oslo, Norway

We describe using transcranial Doppler (TCD) monitoring of the cerebral hemodynamic changes caused by ventricular fibrillation (VF) during cardiac surgery.

Methods and Findings: A 73-year-old man developed VF, which lasted for two minutes and 24 seconds, during coronary artery bypass grafting (CABG). Surgery was performed «off-pump» without cardioplegia and a heart-lung-machine. Continuous TCD monitoring of the left middle cerebral artery (MCA) was performed throughout the operation. A cerebral MRI examination and an extensive neuropsychological evaluation were also performed both before and three months after surgery. This was part of another on-going study regarding cerebral microemboli and neuropsychologic deficits in CABG.

VF resulted immediately in a dramatic fall to zero in MCA blood flow velocities with only slight fluctuations during the duration of VF. This was followed by a pronounced reactive hyperperfusion that lasted for almost eight minutes. An off-line video recording of the TCD findings will be presented. The patient did not have any neurological deficits and there was no MRI evidence of brain ischemia after surgery. Neuropsychological test results were also similar before and at three months after surgery.

Conclusion: This report clearly demonstrates the value of TCD monitoring during cardiovascular surgery. TCD provides on-line information regarding both cerebral hemodynamic changes and embolization, which allows the surgical team to make appropriate immediate interventions to avoid ischemic brain injury.

83

CAROTID ANGIOPLASTY AND STENTING: ULTRASONOGRAPHIC FOLLOW-UP

G.Orlandi, C.Fioretti, M.Mancuso, *M.Puglioli, *R.Padolecchia, L.Murri
Department of Neurosciences, *Unit of Neuroradiology, Pisa, Italy

Thirty patients (24 males, 6 females) of mean age 68,9 yrs (range 54-79 yrs) underwent 32 percutaneous transluminal angioplasty (PTA) procedures for symptomatic severe carotid stenosis in 27 cases and restenosis in 5 cases. PTA alone and PTA with stent placement were performed in 13 and 19 vessels respectively.

A 24 months (range 18-30 months) ultrasonographic follow-up was carried out to evaluate >50% restenosis and microembolic signals detection in ipsilateral middle cerebral artery.

Three of 32 (9,4%) vessels developed asymptomatic restenosis during the follow-up period. Particularly, restenosis occurred in 2 of 13 (15.4%) vessels treated with PTA alone and in 1 of 19 (5.3%) treated with stent placement. Only two restenosis without stenting produced microembolic signals.

These data suggest that carotid stenting seems a procedure more safe than PTA alone in order to prevent restenosis and embolic events and ultrasonography result an useful tool to carry out a long-term follow-up.

84

THE SURGICAL APPROACH IN TREATMENT OF TRAUMATIC CAVERNOUS-CAROTID FISTULES (CCF)

Ranko Raicevic, Aco Jovicic, Ljubomir Minic*, Ljubo Markovic, Petar Aleksic***, Bratislav Magdic. Department of Neurosurgery*, Department of Neurology, Department of Radiology**, Department of Ophtalmology***, Military Medical Academy, Belgrade, FR Yougoslavia.**

Introduction

In the last decade, endovascular surgery rapidly developed, including methods like embolisation which is the treatment of choice for numerous defects of blood vessel wall, specially for CCF, with ideal aim of fistule closing and restoration of a. carotis interna. Traumatic CCF lead to rapid haemodynamic disorders due to flow shunt between a. carotis interna and cavernous sinus with possible development irreversible damage of endocranial structures including cerebral ischemia due to stel phenomenon accompanied with compresion. Urgent recognition of this problem is of outmost importance.

Methods and results

We represent 4 cases of traumatic CCF (sclopetar war wounds with damage of cavernous sinus wall and a. carotis interna). Diagnosis was based on findings of computerised tomography or magnetic resonance of the brain with angiography performed before and after surgical treatment. All patients were treated according to classical surgical approach after the diagnosis was established.

Surgical treatment consisted of a. carotis interna ligature on the neck (C1) and placing the clips on a.carotis interna intracranial before a. ophtalmica (C3). Control angiography proved exclusion of a.carotis interna till C4 segment from circulation in all cases. All patients were without additional neurological deficit after the surgery and three patients had better neurological status.

Conclusion

We conclude that surgical approach still stands for an important method in treatment of CCF especialy in war situations when modern procedures can not be applied in all cases.

85

PHYSIOLOGICAL LIMITS TO CHANGES IN BLOOD FLOW VELOCITY OVER BOTH MEDIAL CEREBRAL ARTERIES DURING THE FIRST DAYS AFTER CAROTID ENDARTERECTOMY

dr. A. Schaafsma, Dept. of Clin. Neurophysiology, Martini Ziekenhuis Groningen, the Netherlands.

Aim: to document physiological changes in flow velocity over both medial cerebral arteries occurring in 60 patients undergoing carotid endarterectomy (CEA) and to detect deviations from this normal pattern for the early diagnosis of a developing hyperperfusion syndrome.

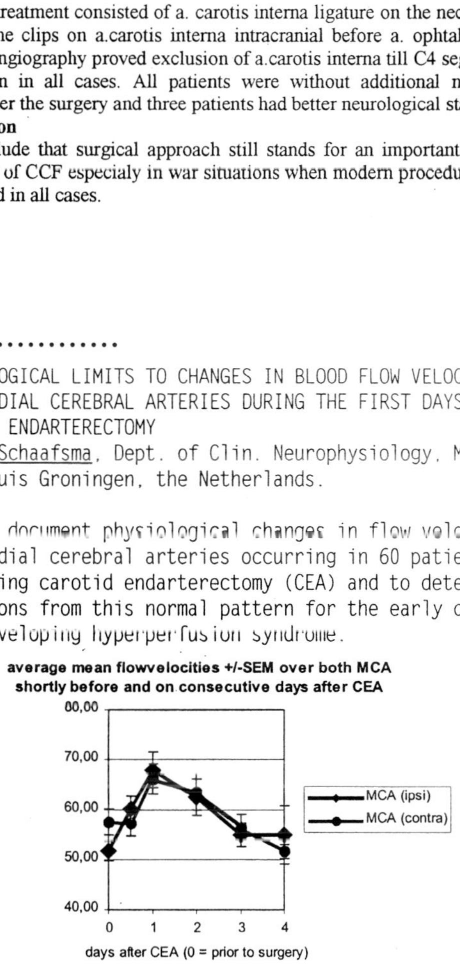

Results: maximal increase in flow velocity on day 1 postCEA. One patient with a continuing increase over day 1 to 3 after CEA. She was treated as an early hyperperfusion syndrome, resulting in a prompt normalization of flow velocities.

Conclusion: awareness of the physiological limits to changes in flow velocity over both MCA following CEA is important for the early detection of a hyperperfusion syndrome.

86

Noninvasive Assessment of CSF Dynamics and Cerebral Venous Outflow in patients with Benign Intracranial Hypertension (BIH).

A.R.Shakhnovich, V.A.Shakhnovich, A.A.Galushkina.
Burdenko Neurosurgery Institute, Moscow, Russia.

Background and Purpose: Venous outflow from surface of the brain is realized by bridging veins which pass the subarachnoid space and fall into superior saggittal sinus. Raise of ICP leads to „cuff constriction" of bridging veins and increase of venous collateral outflow through deep veins and straight sinus. The purpose of this work was noninvasive assessment of CSF dynamics and cerebral venous outflow in BIH.

Material and Methods: The study was carried out on 20 healthy volunteers (HV) (aged 14-52y., m. 9) and 22 patients with BIH (arachnoiditis - 14, endocrine disturbances - 5, superior saggittal sinus thrombosis - 3) (age 11-54 y., m. - 7).
FV in the straight sinus (FVss) was recorded by insonating through occipital window in head up tilt (HUT) test: in horizontal position (HP) of patient, in vertical position (VP) and again in HP. HUT leads to decrease of ICP and returning to HP - to increase of ICP.

Results and Discussion: HP in HV was characterized by normal values of decrease of FVss (mean 16% range 10-22%) and after returning to HP FVss at once came back to initial level (IL). In BIH FVss in HP was increased (mean 52 cm/sec., range 38-84 cm/sec.). In 16 patients with BIH FVss after HUT and returning to HP was significantly higher (up to 72%) or lower (up to 44%) than IL and reached this IL significantly later (mean in 48 sec., range 32-68 sec.)
These changes can be caused by disturbances of CSF dynamics and occlusion of CSF pathways.

Conclusion: HUT allows to assess non-invasively disturbances not only of cerebral venous outflow but also of CSF dynamics in patients with BIH.

87

DOES MICROVASCULAR DOPPLER PREVENT VASCULAR COMPLICATIONS IN CEREBRAL ANEURYSM SURGERY?

R Stendel, A Abo Al Hassan, M Brock

Dept. of Neurosurgery, Benjamin Franklin Medical Center,
Free University of Berlin, Germany

Objective: The outcome of surgical treatment of cerebral aneurysms may be severely impaired by cerebral ischemia or infarction resulting from the inadvertent occlusion of an adjacent vessel by the aneurysm clip or by rebleeding due to incomplete aneurysm occlusion. Therefore it is mandatory to control the surgical result in situ in order to reduce complication rate. The present study was performed to investigate the reliability of microvascular Doppler ultrasonography (MDU) in cerebral aneurysm surgery, and to assess the influence of this method on the surgical procedure.

Methods: Seventy-five patients (19 male, 56 female, mean age 54.8 years, range 22 - 84 years) with 90 saccular cerebral aneurysms were studied. Blood flow velocities in the aneurysmal sac and adjacent vessels were determined by MDU before and after aneurysm clipping. The findings of MDU were analyzed and compared to those of visual inspection and postoperative angiography. It was The cases in which the clip was replaced due to unexpected MDU results were also analyzed.

Results: A relevant stenosis of an adjacent vessel induced by clip positioning that had escaped detection by visual inspection was identified by Doppler ultrasonography in 17 of 90 aneurysms (18.9%). In contrast to the results of visual inspection through the surgical microscope, Doppler ultrasound demonstrated a primarily unoccluded aneurysm in 11 of 90 patients (12.2%). The aneurysm clip was replaced on the basis of the MDU findings in 26 of 90 cases (28.8%). In middle cerebral artery (MCA) aneurysms, the MDU results influenced the surgical procedure in 17 of 44 cases (38.6%). This is statistically significant different as compared to the results in aneurysms of the anterior cerebral artery (5/32; 15.6%) ($p<0.05$).

Conclusion: MDU should be used routinely in cerebral aneurysm surgery, especially in MCA-aneurysms. Postoperative angiography is not necessary whenever there is good visualization of the "working site" and MDU yields clearcut results.

88

ASSESMENT OF CEREBRAL VASOREACTIVITY DURING PHYSICAL EXERCISE

M. Alpaidze. R. Shakarishvili. Z. Metreveli
Sarajishvili Institute of Neurology
Tbilisi, Georgia

Objectives: To evaluate the miogenic vasoreactivity mechanisms in the cerebrovascular regulation.
Subjects and Methods: Seventeen healthy subjects (8-male, 9-female, mean age 29,2±5,4 years) were investigated using TCD at rest and during physical loading. Blood velocity (BV) flow changes in the middle cerebral artery (MCA) and blood pressure (BP) monitoring were carried out. The Resistance Index (RI) and the Pulsative Index (PI) were calculated by analysis of Doppler wave spectrum.
Results: The increase of BP (TT systolic at rest-120±6 mmHg; TTsystolic during exercise-142±9 mmHg p<0,05) affected evident increase of RI and PI values (RI at rest-0,53±0,08, RI during exercise-0,65±0,04 p=0,01. PI at rest-0,95±0,05. PI during exercise-1,2±0,04 p=0.01). Elevation of mean BV in MCA was not statistical significant (deviation from mean BV is by 3,44).
By measuring end-tidal pCO2 levels, it was estimated, that the metabolic regulation mechanism was not responsible for above-mentioned changes.
Conclusion: Physiological miogenic mechanism of vasoreactivity response during physical exercise implies the elevation of RI and PI indexes. This phenomenon is considerable for definition vasoreactivity abnormalities in different neurological disorders.

89

IMPAIRED ADAPTATION OF THE CEREBRAL BLOOD FLOW TO HEAD-UP TILT IN THE ELDERLY

S. Castellani*, I. Carobbi**, N. Boni *, V. Corsoni *, C. Zeloni *, F. Battaglia *, G.F. Gensini *, G. Masotti **
Dipartimento di area critica medica e chirurgica -*Sez. Clinica Medica Generale e Cardiologia; ** Sez. Gerontologia Geriatria e Clinica Urologica; University of Florence, Italy

Orthostatic hypotension syncope and fainting are highly prevalent in the elderly and occur more frequently in the old than in young subjects. The onset of symptoms during prolonged standing may be the consequence of a transient reduction of blood supply to the brain caused by a defect in autoregulation. The aim of this study was to evaluate whether the characteristics of cerebral autoregulation in the orthostatic position (head-up tilt table test - HUT) in the elderly are different with respect to the young. 10 young volunteers (5 men, 5 women aged 21 to 31 yrs - mean 24,5) and 10 healthy elderly (5 men and 5 women; aged 60 to 69 yrs, mean 64,5) have been studied. They were all non-smokers, had a BMI <27, and were not offspring of diabetic or hypertensive patients. Cerebral hemodynamics was studied with transcranial Doppler (Multidop x 4, DWL) by continuous monitoring of the mean velocity (Vm) in the middle cerebral artery (MCA) through the temporal windows by two 2 MHz probes. Arterial blood pressure (Finapres) and CO_2 (Datex Normocap CO_2 monitor) were simultaneously recorded. After laying in the supine position for a 30 minute baseline stabilization period all subjects remained for 20 minutes in a standing position (70° HUT) and subsequently laid supine until all hemodynamic variables had reverted to baseline. HUT significantly reduced arterial blood pressure only in the elderly (-8,5% at peak, vs.baseline, p<0,02 in the elderly; -3,01% at peak, vs. baseline, p= NS in the young). In the elderly, orthostatic stimulation caused a significant drop in Vm in both MCAs during the whole observation (p<0.05 with ANOVA). The reduction peaked at the first 30s observation (-11%; p<0.005 vs baseline) and then remained significantly lower until the end (-2%; p<0.001 vs.baseline). The effects of head-up tilt test on cerebral hemodynamics indicate that the adaptation of the systemic and cerebral circulation to prolonged orthostatic position is impaired in the elderly. Indeed the HUT induced blood pressure reduction was associated in the elderly with a decrease in cerebral blood flow evidenced by the drop in MCA mean velocity. This impairement may explain the higher prevalence of symptomatic orthostatic hypotension observed in the elderly.

90

NEUROPSYCHOLOGICAL AND TRANSCRANIAL DOPPLER (TCD) - MEASURED HEMODYNAMIC CONSEQUENCES IN ESSENTIAL HYPERTENSION

G. Csáti[1], L. Csiba[1], A. Valikovics[1], M. Andrejkovics[1]

Dept. of Neurology (1) and Dept. of Psychiatry (2), University of Debrecen, Faculty of Medicine, Debrecen, Hungary

Background and Purpose: Cerebral vasculature, and cognitive performance changes were found even in complication-free hypertensives. The purpose of the study was to examine wether TCD-assessed selective circulatory changes evoked by cognitive, motor and chemical stimuli has different patterns in untreated hypertensive patients and in normal volunteers.
Methods: 10 right-handed normal volunteers and 11 right-handed untreated, complication-free hypertensives were examined. Subjects performed a battery of breath holding, finger movement, attention, memory, and psychomotor speed tasks. During testing, flow velocities in the left and right middle cerebral artery (**MCA**) were measured continuously by two transcranial Doppler probes fixed with a headband. Blood pressures were also monitored by a Finapres device.
Results: Significant differences between hypertensives and controls were observed in the moment of maximum and minimum flow velocity value in both MCA-s (p=0,007 and 0,045) during the breath holding task, relative velocity changes in both MCA-s (p=0,008 left, and 0,030 right) during finger movement task, moment of minimum velocity value in left MCA (p=0,007) during an attention test, the vasomotor range parameter (**VMR**) of both MCA-s during a discrimination task (p=0,002 left and 0,0001 rigth side), maximum velocity in the left MCA during a fluency task (p=0,030), VMR of the left MCA during a verbal memory task (p=0,040). Neuropsychological performance difference was observed on visual discrimination task (p=0,037). Side-to-side and gender-related MCA velocity differences during tasks were also found.
Conclusions: MCA velocity and cognitive differences were found between hypertensives and normal volunteers. Confirmation of these findings on larger groups needs further investigations.

91

Dynamic cerebral autoregulation assessed from spontaneous blood pressure transients is impaired after acute stroke.

M Blake[1], S Dawson[1], P Eames[1], R Panerai[2], J Potter[1].
Divisions of Medicine for the Elderly[1] and Medical Physics[2], University of Leicester, England

Introduction: Dynamic cerebral autoregulation (CA) can be estimated from spontaneous changes in blood pressure (BP) found in baseline recording without inducing BP changes. No co-operation is required from the subject, discomfort is minimised and there is no change induced from any external stimulus in sympathetic/vagal activity or in pCO2 levels.
Methods: We studied 69 CT diagnosed ischaemic stroke patients (aged 39-89) within 72 hours of ictus and 98 normal controls (aged 34-81). Cerebral blood flow velocity, measured in both middle cerebral arteries using transcranial Doppler ultrasound (TCD), non-invasive beat-to-beat measurements of arterial BP, ECG and transcutaneous pCO2 levels were recorded over two 5 minute periods under conditions of minimal external stimuli during supine rest.
Results: Dynamic CA assessed using pressor transients (spontaneous BP increases ≥5 mmHg) was significantly reduced in stroke patients compared to controls (ARIs 3.6±2.4 vs 4.6±2.1 respectively, p=0.01). A similar trend was seen using spontaneous depressor changes (ARIs 4.1±2.1 vs 4.7±2.2 for stroke patients and controls respectively, p=0.08). A small difference was found in the magnitude of spontaneous pressor BP transients between stroke patients and controls (9.7±3.1 mmHg vs 8.4±2.5 mmHg respectively, p=0.01) and in the rate of BP change (3.8±1.9 mmHg/s vs 3.2±1.3 mmHg/s respectively, p=0.04). In the stroke patients no ARI differences were found between the stroke and non-stroke hemispheres. Multiple linear regression showed the ARI differences between the two groups were accounted for by group and unrelated to size or rate of BP transients or baseline BP levels. There was no significant difference in the magnitude or rate of BP change in the spontaneous depressor stimuli.
Conclusions: The study has demonstrated that acute ischaemic stroke is associated with a global impairment of dynamic CA as assessed using spontaneous pressor BP transients.

92

Investigation of brain function is hypertension. A review. Simultaneous SPECT and transcranial Doppler examination during acetazolamide provocation in non treated hypertensive patients

Andrea Ficzere M.D., László Csiba M.D.,
University of Debrecen, Department of Neurology

Functional and morphological abnormalities due to hypertension could be detected by CT, MRI, transcranial Doppler ultrasound, PET and SPECT on neurologically symptom-free patients. The single or combined application of these techniques reveal different aspects of parenchymal or vascular impairment in hypertension. The advantages and disadvantages of different imaging techniques are reviewed and compared. The relatively simple, non-invasive transcranial Doppler (alone or combined with neuropsychological observations) could be recommended for screening and follow up of hypertensive patients and seems to be a promising tool for evaluation of efficacy of antihypertensive therapy.

In the second part of the poster we summarize the preliminary results of an acetazolamide stimulation in hypertensive patients done simultaneously by transcranial Doppler and single photon emission tomography. According to the literature the of rCBF of SPECT and TCD have coincided in 91 % of the hemispheres. Since the study is in progress, the numerical results will be available just at the time of the congress. The preliminary results suggests a slight global decrease in the cerebral blood flow with the same change in the velocity in the MCA.

93

DURATION OF INTRACRANIAL VASODILATION FOLLOWING ARTERIAL INJECTION OF VERAPAMIL

A. Hartmann [1,2], A. Faulstich [2], W.L. Young [1], N. Ostapkovich [1], S. Trocio [1], H. Mast [1,3], D.H. Duong[1], J.P. Mohr [1]

[1] New York Presbyterian Hospital, New York, US, [2] Universtätsklinikum Benjamin Franklin, Berlin, German, [3] Berufsgenossenschaftliche Klinik Bergmannstrost, Halle, Germany

Introduction: Intraarterial injection of verapamil is used to prevent vasospasm during neurointerventional treatment of intracranial arteries. However, the time course of the vasodilatory effect has not been described. Transcranial Doppler (TCD) is used for monitoring intracranial blood flow, and increase of TCD mean flow velocity (MV) reflects vasodilation distal to the insonation site.

Methods: The 7 patients (5 female, mean age 36, SD 14.7 years) of the New York Presbyterian Hospital Vasodilator Study were assessed. A total dose of 4.5 mg verapamil was given as a constant infusion over 4.5 minutes at a rate of 1mg/minute via an arterial catheter into the distal internal carotid artery. Vasodilation was measured by TCD using an EME Pioneer with a handheld pulsed-wave 2 MHz probe. From a transtemporal approach the M1-segment of the middle cerebral artery was insonated at a depth of 50 mm. Mean MV increase of all patients was analyzed and taken to document the vasodilatory effect of verapamil. Time to maximum MV and mean MV increase at the end of infusion were calculated.

Results: All patients responded to the intraarterial infusion with an increase of MV: Baseline MV was 61 cm/s (SD 22 cm/s). Maximum MV of 79 cm/s (SD 21 cm/s) was observed after a mean of 128 seconds (SD 63 seconds). At the end of infusion after 4.5 minutes MV had almost returned to baseline (66 cm/s, SD 20 cm/s). No effect on systemic arterial pressure was observed.

Conclusions: The vasodilatory effect of intracranial arterial injection of verapamil is of short duration. Possible explanations are (1) slower relaxation of proximal vessels compared with distal arteriolar vessels and (2) rapid pharmacologic offset after arterial injection without systemic effect. This should be noted if considered for use in the management of vasospasm during intracranial interventional procedures.

94

IMPORTANT ROLE OF TRANSCRANIAL DOPPLER IN SUBARACHNOIDAL HAEMORRHAGE IN REDUCING A NUMBER OF FALSE-NEGATIVE ANGIOGRAPHY RESULTS

H. Hećimović, V. Vargek-Solter, M. Bošnjak, T. Breitenfeld, V. Vuković, V. Demarin, Department of Neurology, University Hospital, Zagreb, Croatia

Subarachnoidal haemorrhage usually occurs following a rupture of saccular aneurysm. The rupture of aneurysm presents an urgent diagnostic problem and following admission of the patients with subarachnoidal haemorrhage we performed lumbar puncture, CT scan and, if necessary, cerebral angiography. In this work we analyzed the patients admitted to our hospital in the ten years period, i.e. before and after introducing transcranial doppler (TCD) to detect spasm of cerebral arteries.

In 1998, 31 patients were hospitalized because of non-traumatic subarachnoidal haemorrhage, and 27 patients were admitted with subarachnoid haemorrhage in 1988. CT scan confirmed the diagnosis of subarachnoidal haemorrhage in 83% of patients admitted in 1998 and in 92% of patients in 1988, respectively. Further on, cerebral angiography showed an aneurysm in 81% with positive CT scan in 1998, and in 55% of patients in 1988, respectively. From these results, it appears that there were significantly more patients in 1998 with visible aneurysm on angiography, than ten years earlier. This was to great extent due to the use of TCD for daily monitoring of cerebral vasospasm and, therefore, better timing for angiography. Vasospasm on angiography was a major complaint of radiologists in 1988. When we further analyzed 6 patients from 1998 in whom angiography showed no aneurysm, 4 of them had cerebral vasospasm on transcranial doppler, and this may be the reason they had false-negative angiography.

In conclusion TCD is a valuable non-invasive tool for diagnostics of cerebral circulation and should be used for daily monitoring of cerebral vasospasm to decrease a number of false-negative angiography results. In addition to TCD, we found a marked effect of continuous intravenous application of nimodipine in prevention and reducing cerebral vasospasm, so decreasing possibility of early ishaemic stroke while waiting for surgery.

95

ILOPROST INDUCED COUNTER-STEAL IN SUBACUTE MIDDLE CEREBRAL ARTERY INFARCTION

O. Hoffmann, S. Schreiber, H. Obrig, A. Villringer, J.R. Weber, J.M. Valdueza

Neurologische Klinik der Charité, Humboldt-Universität, D-10098 Berlin

Background— The effects of iloprost, a vasodilatory prostaglandin I_2 analogue, on human regional cerebral blood flow (rCBF) have not been studied in healthy subjects or after stroke.

Case Description— We report transcranial Doppler (TCD) and near infrared spectroscopy (NIRS) findings in a 68 year old female patient who was treated with i.v. iloprost for limb ischemia three weeks after left-hemispheric stroke. While no acute effect of iloprost could be demonstrated in the unaffected hemisphere, mean blood flow velocities in the middle cerebral artery (MCA) on the side of infarction increased to 150 % of baseline during infusion. NIRS revealed a simultaneous increase of [total Hb] and [oxy-Hb] and a decrease of [deoxy-Hb] on the affected side only. CO_2 reactivity of the mean blood flow velocity was normal in the right MCA but abolished in the left MCA.

Conclusion—Impaired CO_2 reactivity on the side of infarction suggests that the counter-steal phenomenon is caused by a disturbed metabolic coupling of the rCBF which may counteract the vasodilatory effect of iloprost in the normal cerebral circulation.

96

Hofmann-RP*, Steinmeier-R**

A COMPARISON OF CEREBRAL AUTOREGULATION TESTS IN PRACTICE

* Department of Neurology, Chemnitz Medical Center, Chemnitz, Germany
** Department of Neurosurgery, Technical University of Dresden, Germany

Objective: Knowledge about cerebral autoregulation in patients with traumatic brain injury (TBI) or subarachnoid haemorrhage (SAH) may be useful to influence patient's therapy management.
Methods: Continuous monitoring of arterial blood pressure, intracranial pressure and flow velocity in middle cerebral artery as well as 4 different bedside autoregulation tests (altogether 411 tests) were performed in 13 of patients with severe TBI or a SAH (HUNT & HESS scale > 3). Results of 107 cuff deflation tests, 112 transient hyperaemic response tests, 131 orthostatic hypotension tests and 61 tests using an artificial arterial-blood-pressure-triggering by forced ventilation were compared. For validation, sensitivity, specificity and diagnostic score for both pairs of cerebral autoregulation tests as well as all cerebral autoregulation tests together were calculated.
Results: Only a minor agreement was found. Comparing all tests together, an agreement was found in 4,4 %, whereas contrary statements were found in 40 %, i.e. approximately 1 corresponding statement comes to 4 contrary. In paired comparison, no superiority was found. Cuff deflation and orthostatic hypotension were noticed to be relatively sensitive (Se = 0,733) and specific (Sp = 0,667) resulting in the highest diagnostic score of 140 %.
Discussion: We found a low predictive reliability for cerebral autoregulation at a certain moment or further course by means of these tests. Orthostatic hypotension turned out to have a good prevalence as a multifactoral test with a high threshold and a wide intermediate zone between predicted impaired and normal cerebral autoregulation. Probably a better evaluation of these tests is possible by comparison with imaging methods, i.e. Xenon-CCT, SPECT or PET.

97

Hofmann-RP*, Steinmeier-R**

TRANSIENT HYPERAEMIC RESPONSE TEST AND ITS CLINICAL PRACTICABILITY

* Department of Neurology, Chemnitz Medical Center, Chemnitz, Germany
** Department of Neurosurgery, Technical University Dresden, Germany

Objective: Transient Hyperaemic Response Test (THRT) is an easy to perform bedside autoregulation tool without sophisticated technical and personal effort (introduced by GILLER et al. in 1991). It was examined for its practicability in clinical routine.
Methods: In 13 adults with traumatic brain injury or subarachnoid haemorrhage, 99 THRT were performed. In each test, averaging of 3 consecutive runs was performed.
Results: Stochastic influences resulting from the signal itself as well as deterministic influences by physiological parameters and way of test performance were found to lead to pitfalls in interpretation of THRT. Carrying out an averaging over 4 consecutive heart cycles (in order to ascertain mean flow velocity in middle cerebral artery (FV_{mean}) before and after carotid compression) as well as paying attention to wave phenomena of transcranial Doppler signal, CPP dependency of FV as well as depth and duration of carotid compression will lead to a different test results for cerebral autoregulation in 23,2 % and to a reduction of standard deviation of averaged FV_{mean} out of each run of 57,5 %. In comparison to other bedside autoregulation tests (cuff deflation, orthostatic hypotension and artificial arterial-blood-pressure-triggering by forced ventilation), and a higher specificity for a disturbed cerebral autoregulation was found.
Discussion: Validity of modified THRT seems to be small in comparison to other bedside autoregulation tests. Diagnostic score in comparison to cuff deflation test was 46 %, to autoregulation test by forced ventilation 14,2 % and to orthostatic hypotension 45,2 %. One-parametric approach, single threshold and leakage of an intermediate zone between normal and impaired cerebral autoregulation should be discussed to be the reason.

98

Bauhuf-C*, Hofmann-RP**, Steinmeier-R***, Hübner-U*

EVALUATION OF CEREBRAL AUTOREGULATION IN HEALTHY VOLUNTEERS USING CROSS-CORRELATION ANALYSIS

* Department of Neurosurgery, Faculty of Clinical Medicine Mannheim, University of Heidelberg, Germany
** Department of Neurology, Chemnitz Medical Center, Chemnitz, Germany
*** Department of Neurosurgery, Technical University of Dresden, Germany

Objective: In a recent study, cross-correlation (CC) analysis was applied on digital recordings of arterial blood pressure (ABP), intracranial pressure (ICP) and intracranial blood flow velocity (FV). A lack of time delay and positive correlation of slow oscillations between these parameters was interpreted as impaired autoregulatory response, whereas significant time delay and negative correlation was regarded as an indicator for preserved cerebral autoregulation.
Methods: In order to test this hypothesis, we performed CC analysis on recordings of ABP and FV in 17 healthy volunteers. Non-invasive continuous ABP was recorded using a radial tonometric device, FV measurements were taken from bilateral middle cerebral arteries (MCA). Signals were sampled at resting horizontal position. CC was calculated offline after a lowpass filtering procedure.
Results: In all cases, spontaneous slow oscillations of ABP and FV could be detected by means of spectral analysis. In the time domain analysis of slow oscillations, *mean time delay* (T) for CC[ABP FV_{left}] was 6.45 s ± 2.1, CC[ABP FV_{right}] was 6.09 s ± 1.8 and CC[ABP FV] was 6.29 s ± 1.93, *mean CC-coefficient* was -0.33 s ± 0.17 for the left, -0.36 s ± 0.09 for the right side and -0.35 s ± 0.14 for both sides together (CC[FV_{right} FV_{left}]), all confirmed by a data cluster analysis.
Discussion: The observed time course of ABP and FV signals agrees well with results from former studies on the dynamic nature of cerebral autoregulation. Since CC analysis is applicable without any external triggering of ABP changes, this study provides further evidence that this method is potentially useful as a bedside tool for continuous cerebral autoregulation monitoring.

99

ROLE OF CEREBRAL VASOMOTION IN THE SPONTANEOUS FLUCTUATIONS OF CEREBRAL BLOOD FLOW VELOCITY

H.H.Hu, MD, T.B.J.Kuo, MD, PhD & W.J.Wong, MD
Section of Cerebrovascular Disease, Veteran General Hospital-Taipei, Taipei, Taiwan, R.O.C.

Background and purpose : In order to explore the mechanism of spontaneous fluctuations in cerebral blood velocity, beat-to-beat variability in cerebrovascular resistance (CVR), evaluated by resistance index (RI) and pulsatility index (PI), and its relationship to mean velocity (MV) of the middle cerebral artery were analyzed in frequency-domain.
Methods : There were 10 normal volunteers with a mean age (± SD) of 32±5.7 years. Five-min flow velocity signals at supine rest in the daytime were recorded using transcranial Doppler sonography. Spectral and transfer function analyses of percentile CVR and MV variability were performed by fast Fourier transform.
Results : All CVR indexes exhibited significant variability which was around 6%-10% of the mean value. Over 80% of CVR variability was confined to the 3 frequency ranges, designated as high- (0.15-0.4 Hz, HF), low- (0.04-0.15 Hz, LF) and very low-frequency (0.016-0.04 Hz, VLF) components. PI had a greater variability than RI; however, the frequency distribution of variability was similar for those two CVR indexes. All of the HF, LF and VLF components of CVR exhibited high coherence (linearity) with those of MV. Transfer function analysis of the CVR-MV relationship revealed that the transfer magnitude was near 1 and the transfer phase was close to 180 degree in the VLF and LF ranges. The transfer phase in HF range was broadly scattered.
Conclusions : The cerebral vasomotion may play a major role in the generation of VLF and LF variability of cerebral blood flow velocity. Another mechanism may be responsible for the HF variability.

100

TRANSCRANIAL DOPPLER SONOGRAPHY WITH FUNCTIONAL TESTS FOR DIAGNOSIS OF TIA IN THE VERTEBRO-BASILAR SYSTEM

V.I. Kalashnikov
Ukrainian SRI of Clinical and Experimental Neurology and Psychiatry, Kharkiv, Ukraine

Aim of the work: To investigate a state of the cerebra vascular reactivity (CVR) in patients with TIA in th vertebro-basilar system (VBS) by transcranial Dopple sonography (TCD) with functional tests such as hypercapnic orthostatic (OT), and rotation probes (RP).
Methods: 48 middle aged patients were examined. 26 patient had TIAs due to cervical spondyloarthrosis (CS) and 2 patients had TIAs due to arterial hypertension (AH).
Results: The blood flow velocity asymmetry (25-30%) i vertebral arteries (VAs) occurred in 23.6% of AH patients an 41.9% of CS patients. A hyperreactivity on CO_2 was pointe out in 33.2% of AH patients and 11.8% of CS patients; a hypo reactivity on CO_2 was pointed out in 20.7% and 8.1% o patients respectively. The hyperreactivity on OT was foun out in 28.4% of AH patients and 38.5% of CS patients; a abnormal reactivity on OT was found out in 5.1% and 12.8% o patients respectively. Under conditions of RP 20.3% of A patients and 36.4% of CS patients had a spasm in one of VAs 12.1% and 19.6% of patients respectively had a spasm in VA and basilar arteries (BAs), and a hypoperfusion in VAs wa observed in 14.1% and 25.1% of patients respectively.
Conclusions: TIA development in VBS in patients with CS i connected with VAs and BAs regional dysgemias enhanced by R and resulting in a disorder of neurogenic brain blood flo regulation. Appearance of TIAs in VBS in patients with AH i associated with CVR disorders on all levels and wit dysfunction of the humoral metabolic mechanism first of all.

101

THE PROGNOSTIC VALUE OF SERIAL TCD-EXAMINATIONS AFTER CARDIO-PULMONARY RESUSCITATION

[1]Christof Klötzsch, [1]C.Jacke, [2]O.Popescu, [1]J.Noth
Depts.of Neurology [1]RWTH Aachen, [2]Klinikum Saarbrücken, Germany

Background: The decrease of cerebral flow velocity and increase of the resistance index (RI) during the first days after cardio-pulmonary resuscitation (CPR) was described previously. The aim of this study was to estimate the potential of transcranial Doppler sonography (TCD) to predict the clinical outcome of patients after CPR on the basis of intracranial flow velocity changes.
Methods: Thirty-one consecutive patients (7 women, 24 men; aged 17 to 78 years) who survived cardio-pulmonary arrest were involved. Serial TCD-examinations (MDX-4, DWL, Germany) of the large intracranial vessels were performed 4, 8, 16, 24 and 72 hours after CPR. Ventilation parameters (pH, pO2, pCO2) and hemodynamic parameters (heart rate, blood pressure) were recorded together with the TCD-parameters.
Results: Twenty patients (group 1.) either died (n=19) within 8±10 days or remained in a vegetative state (n=1). Eleven patients (group 2.) survived asymptomatic or had minimal neurological deficits. Postanoxic myoclonus was observed in 10 patients (50%) of group 1. and one patient (9%) of group 2. The neuron specific enolase (NSE) level in plasma ranged from 22-1242 mg/l in group 1. and from 9-29 mg/l in group 2. A comparison of the flow velocities in the middle cerebral artery (MCA) 4 and 24 hours after CPR revealed an increase of the peak systolic velocities of 10% in group 1. and 67% in group 2. while diastolic velocities increased 17% in group 1. and 108% in group 2. Similar changes were found in the remaining intracranial vessels (anterior/posterior cerebral artery, basilar artery).
Conclusions: This TCD-study revealed a significant increase of systolic and diastolic flow velocity within the first 24 hours in patients who survive cardio-pulmonary arrest without severe neurological deficits. Independent from medication and ventilation parameters serial TCD-examinations are able to predict early the clinical outcome in patients after CPR.

102

ARTERIAL PREASSURE FLUCTUATION AS A RESULT OF STENOSIS OR OCCLUSION OF CAROTID ARTERIES IN COLOR DOPPLER MEASUREMENTS.

E.Kudybka-Glownia;J.Siejka-Jurenczyk
Neurology dept.Municipal Hospital
Katowice-Murcki,Poland

Hypertension is serious risk factor and sometimes pathogenetic factor of cerebral blood flow (CBF) disorders which occurs suddenly.The signifi cant thing is correlation between treatment-resistant hypertension of unknown origin and stenosis of carotid arteries (common or/and internal CCA or ICA).

A group of 84 patients with violently fluctuating hypertension (RR up to 220/100) of unknown origin had been examined.Patients suffered from headaches, dizziness,numbness or paraesthesia and sometimes visual disorders;neurological examination usually showed hemilateral or bilateral pyramid symptoms (transient or fixed).Such tests as Color Doppler measurement,lipid,cholesterol levels and coagulating factors had been performed invariably.
Disorders of CBF concerning especially right hemisphere of brain were found out in all cases. Atherosclerotic plates visualised mostly within the division of CCA and ICA bulb caused stenosis in them up to 30% in 47% of patients , 30-50% in 33% of patients , more than 50% in 16% of cases and occlusion of the vessel in 4% of patients.
Described abnormalities occured bilaterally in the group of 40% of patients, in 41% of cases concerned mostly right ICA and in 19% of cases - left ICA.It is considerably important that despite anticlot treatment the coagulating factors were high(INR 1,5) and lipids level was increased in the group of 39% of patients.

Finally,pharmacological menagement of CBF disorders without agressive decreasing of hypertension caused both-withdrawal of neurological symptoms and stabilization of arterial preassure at the level 150-160/80-90.

103

TRANSCRANIAL STRESS-DOPPLEROGRAPHY TO ASSESS CEREBRAL AUTOREGULATION

V.P. Kulikov, N.L. Doronina
Altai State Medical University, Barnaul, Russia

Our study was undertaken to check the possibilities of using light physical exercises (PE) to assess autoregulation of cerebral blood flow. The premise for it was the fact that light PE changes central hemodynamics and blood pressure (BP).
35 healty volunteers and 50 patients with damages of internal carotid arteries (ICA) as aterosclerotic stenosis or pathological kinking have been studied. All subjects were examined at scanner «Spectra Masters» (USA). Peak systolic velocity (Vps), end diastolic velocity (Ved), time average maximal velocity of blood flow (TAMX) and the indexes of vascular resistance (RI and PI) were measured in the middle cerebral artery (MCA). Minute volume of left ventricle, heart index were measured by echodopplercardiography; BP according to Korotkov. The indexes were fixed at rest and after PE which was performed as squatings for 30 sec.
The results have showen that the increase of Vps to 44,9%, Ved to 23,3%, TAMX - 32,0%, RI - 15,5% and PI to 29,1% (p<0,05) in the MCA was a steady response of brain blood circulation to light PE. The response of Vps. TAMX to PE in subjects with damages of ICA was less marked comparing with heathy subjects; response of Ved was to not found. A correlatation of cerebral and central hemodynamics which differed in patients and heathy subjects was established. Interconnected and different changes of systemic and peripherical cerebral vascular resistance during PE might be considered as the reflection of cerebral hemodynamics autoregulation. On the basis of the data obtained 2 types of the calculation of cerebral autoregulation indexes are establisted. The first method is based on the calcullation relative changes of cerebrovascular resistanse in MCA. It is referreed to as the index of cerebral autoregulation (ICAR). ICAR was 2,5 times higher in healthy men than in those with stenoses in ICA (p<0,01). The second index was obtained by the methods of discriminant analysis and marked as the index of cerebral autoregulation condition (CARC). The autoregulation is preserved in the positive meaning of CARC while in its negative meaning CARC is disturbed.

104

FUNCTIONAL STATE OF BRAIN IN CHILDREN WITH PATOLOGICAL KINKING OF INTERNAL CAROTID ARTERIES

V.P. Kulikov, J.V. Smirnova, K.V. Smirnov, V.I. Kling
Altai State Medical University, Barnaul, Russia

To determine hemodynamic importance of pathological kinking (PK) of internal carotid arteries (ICA) in children the indexes of blood flow in middle cerebral arteries (MCA) as well as functional state of brain were studied. 35 children (aged 7-14) having according to color dupplex scanning (CDS) PK of ICA were examined. Group A composed of 16 children with bilateral PK of ICA. Group B composed of 19 children with unilateral PK. CDS of neck vessles as well as MCA were performed using scanning «Spectra Masters» (USA). The functional state of brain was assessed according to the results of electroencephalogram (EEG), to visual and cognitive evoked potentials as well as to magnetic stimulation of pyramidal tract with the help of stimulator «Magstim 200» (England).

It has been established that PK of ICA in children was characterized by a marked turbulence of blood flow at the site of PK with increasing of peak systolic velocity of blood flow (PS). Besides, the reduction of PS in both MCA was found in group A. But in group B it was stated at the site of PK localization. The disturbance of bioelectric brain activity (BBA) as diffuse changes of EEG of different degrees were registered in 15 out 16 subjects with bilateral PK of ICA; epileptiform activity (EA) was determined in 7 subjects. Bilateral disfunction of visual nerves, the reduction of operative memory volume and decreasing of motoric cortex (MC) excitability toward magnetic stimuli were marked in all patients of the group A. In the case of unilateral PK of ICA (group B) the changes of BBA as diffuse alterations of EEG were registered in 17 out of 19 subjects. Focal EA at the site of the damaged artery according to EEG data was registered in 8. The damage of visual nerve at the site of pathological activity was found in 17. The reduction of operative memory volume as well as the decreasing of excitability of MC toward magnetic stimuli were found in 16 out 19 of children. Thus, PK of ICA in children is acompanied by the marked damages of functional brain state as the reduction of blood flow to MCA, by diffuse alterations and EA at EEG, disfunction of visual nerves, reduction of operative memory volume as well as by decreasing of MC excitablity.

105

EVALUATION OF CEREBROVASCULAR REACTIVITY IN CHILDREN WITH HEADACHE.

Kwieciński J, Biernawska J, Kapustecki J, Pierzchała K.
Department of Neurology Silesian School of Medicine, Zabrze, Poland

Headache occurs in a half of school-children population while migraine in about 5%. Migraine attacks occur with changes of cerebral arteries lumen. The aim of our study was to estimate Cerebrovascular Reactivity (CVR) in relation of sex, type of headache and neurological status determined by EEG and CT results. Material and methods: the study group consisted of 20 children (11 male, 9 female) of mean age 13,25±3,1 yr. Half of them suffered from migraine headaches, another part from non-migraine headaches. In all subjects neurological examination, EEG, brain CT and TCD was done. TCD examination, including evaluation BFV and PI of both MCA's and evaluation of CVR (percentage ratio of BFV in MCA to pCO_2 decrease after 30 s hyperventilation) was performed using TC 2020 Pioneer (EME) and capnograph Datex (Normocap). Obtained results were compared to control group consisted of 32 age-matched, healthy subject. Results and conclusions: BFV of both MCA's and CVR were significantly higher in children with headache compared to controls ($p<0,05$, $p<0,001$ respectively). Type of headache, EEG and CT results didn't revealed its influence on results of TCD examination. Significantly correlation ($r=0,689$) between BFV and CVR in examined children with headache was observed. Excessive value of CVR and hyperkinetic circulation resulting in disturbance of regional blood flow probably play role in pathogenesis in childhood headache.

106

CEREBRAL BLOOD FLOW IN HYPERTHYROIDISM
- Transcranial Doppler Study -

Y.S. Lee, J.S. Jeon*, B.K. Kim**, S.H. Park
Department of Neurology
Seoul Municipal Boramae Hospital & Eulji General Hospital**
Department of Internal Medicine, Eulji General Hospital*

Hyperdynamic cardiovascular changes are well defined in hyperthyroidism. Peripheral blood flow is increased by the thyroid hormone-mediated reduction of systemic vascular resistance. However, cerebral blood flow changes in hyperthyroidism and the effect of thyroid hormone on cerebral vessels have not been known well. Using TCD, we try to reveal the abnormal cerebral blood flow changes and its physiological implication in hyperthyroidism. Thirty-one consecutive patients diagnosed as Graves' disease aged 20 to 40 years (M:F=8:23, 32.8±7.4 years) and 108 age-matched healthy controls (M:F=45:63, 30.4±5.9 years) were prospectively included. Severity of hyperthyroidism was graded as euthyroidism (free T4 < 2.0), mild hyperthyroidism (2.0 ≤ free T4 < 3.0), and severe hyperthyroidism (free T4 ≥ 3.0). TCD was performed to measure the mean flow velocity (MFV) and pulsatility index (PI) of 11 intracranial and 4 extracranial vessels. Elevated MFV (≥2 SD), asymmetry of MFV of middle (≥35%) or anterior cerebral arteries (≥50%), and elevated hemispheric index (≥3.0) were regarded as abnormal. Systolic BP (130 mm Hg vs. 123 mm Hg), pulse rate (80/min vs. 73/min) and frequency of TCD abnormality (45% vs. 10%) was significantly increased in patients. Compared to control, MFV was elevated in intracranial as well as in extracranial vessels ($p<0.01$). MFV was highest in severe hyperthyroidism, while lowest in euthyroidism ($p<0.05$). PI value, influenced by several factors including vascular resistance, was increased in intracranial vessels ($P<0.05$). These preliminary results suggest that cerebral blood flow is increased in proportion to the severity of hyperthyroidism. Cerebral blood flow seems to be mainly influenced by hyperdynamic cardiovascular status rather than the reduced vascular resistance in hyperthyroidism. This physiologic character of cerebral vessels requires* further verification.

107

CORRELATION BETWEEN INVASIVE CBF MEASUREMENTS AND VENOUS AND ARTERIAL TRANSCRANIAL DUPLEX MEASUREMENTS

Mursch K[1], Buhre W[2], Kazmair S[2], Radke K[2], Al-Soufi S[2], Behnke- Mursch J[3]
Depts. Of Neurosurgery[1], and Anaesthesiology[2], Georg-August- University Göttingen, Dept. of Neurosurgery, Zentralklinik Bad Berka[3], Germany.

Objective: To evaluate the possibility of cerebral blood flow (CBF) estimations by venous Doppler investigations.

Methods: Invasive CBF mesurements were performed in 15 patients after subarachnoid hemorrhage (SAH) or traumatic brain injury (TBI), during normoventilation and hyperventilation, using the modified Kety- Schmidt- method. Simultaneously, mean flow velocities in the middle cerebral artery (MCA), the basal vein (BVR) and the internal carotid artery (ICA) were performed using TCCS. 40 valid measurement during variation of PaCO2 were performed.

Results: Multiple regression analysis revealed a significant ß between CBF and BVR velocities only.

Conclusion: The lack of muscular regulation mechanisms may lead to a better representation of CBF by venous TCD or TCCS compared to arteries.

108

Cerebrovascular Response to Head-Up Tilt in Patients with TIAs of Hemodynamic Origin

L. Niehaus, C.H. Nolte, G. Böckeler, B.-U. Meyer
Dept. of Neurology, Charité, Virchow-Klinikum, Berlin, Germany

Transient ischemic attacks (TIAs) of hemodynamic origin can occur in patients with severe stenosis or occlusion of the internal carotid artery (ICA). They are often difficult to identify, since clinical features might resemble those in simple partial seizures or migrainous attacks. Diagnosing hemodynamic compromise in such patients is crucial to start adequate treatment.

We used functional transcranial Doppler sonography (fTCD) to assess the cerebral hemodynamic response to orthostasis in 3 patients with hemodynamic TIAs. One patient presented with transient monocular pain, blurred vision and contralateral limb shaking. Two patients complained of episodes of hypaesthesia or involuntary movements of the arm contralateral to the occluded ICA. Using a bilateral 2-MHz probe holder the mean blood flow velocity (MBFV) in both middle cerebral arteries (MCA) was continuously registered before, during and after 70° head-up tilt.

In healthy volunteers (n=15; aged 42-82 years) MBFV dropped by 11 ± 6 % (mean ± SD) during orthostasis. In patients MBFV dropped by 24 % (range: 17-30%) in the MCA ipsilateral to the ICA occlusion and by 9 % (range: 2-14%) in the MCA contralaterally. Changes in blood pressure and heart rate did not differ between patients and healthy subjects.

Our findings demonstrate an asymmetric cerebral hemodynamic response to orthostasis in patients with TIAs of hemodynamic origin. The marked reduction of MBFV indicate an impaired mechanism of hemodynamic autoregulation in the hemisphere ipsilateral to the occluded ICA. In conclusion tilt-table examination with fTCD might be a useful diagnostic tool in patients with symptomatic ICA occlusion.

109

VINPOCETINE-INDUCED CHANGES IN HEMOGLOBIN CONCENTRATION AND REGIONAL CEREBRAL BLOOD FLOW: A NIRS AND TCD STUDY.

G.Panczel, P.Bönöczk, Z.Nagy
National Stroke Center, Budapest, Hungary

Purpose: Vinpocetine (VP) was suggested to improve cerebral microcirculation by altering hemorheology and vascular resistance. In a placebo -controlled study VP-induced changes in regional cerebral blood flow (rCBF) were assessed by near-infrared spectroscopy (NIRS) and transcranial Doppler sonography (TCD).

Methods and results: We monitored cerebral blood flow velocity (CBFV) and Doppler spectral intensity (DSI) in the middle cerebral arteries (MCA) by TCD in 40 patients with MCA-territory stroke symptoms with relevant infarction on CT, during i.v. infusion of 500 ml Saline alone (placebo group) or with 20 mg VP (VP group). In a consecutive cohort of patients with same inclusion criteria the quantities of different chromophores (Hb=deoxy-hemoglobin, HbO=oxy-hemoglobin, HbT=total hemoglobin i.e. the sum of Hb and HbO) were measured in the frontoparietal region on the side of lesion by NIRS during the same treatment paradigm. Changes in CBFV, DSI and in chromophore quantities (means of first and last 5-min periods of 45-min infusion periods) were compared between groups. Values are given as means$\pm CI_{95}$. DSI showed a significant increase in the treatment group (44.6±7,79 → 70.40±16,50, p=0.005) but not in the placebo group; there were no overt CBFV changes in either groups. All chromophores showed more substantial increase in VP group compared with placebo group (VP group: HbO: −1.01±0.40 → -0.09±1.14 p=0.03; Hb: −0.43±0.23 → -0.32±0.30 p=0.17; HbT: −1.44±0.56 → -0.41±1.13 p=0.01; Placebo group: HbO: -0.95±0.60 → -0.38±0.95 p=0.09; Hb: -0.74±0.53 → -1.00±0.67 p=0.06; HbT -1.69±1.07 → -1.38±1.26 p=0.22). Differences in Hb between groups reached level of statistical significance (p<0.03).

Conclusion: Our data suggest, that increase of rCBF induced by VP outweighs that of placebo. Conventional TCD velocity analysis missed to detect these CBF changes. NIRS monitoring seems to be feasible for the assessment of changes in regional cerebral blood flow.

110

IS DYNAMIC CEREBRAL AUTOREGULATION INFLUENCED BY SYMPATHETIC TONE ?

R.B. Panerai[1], S.L. Dawson[2], J.F. Potter[2]

[1]Depts. Medical Physics and [2]Medicine for the Elderly, University of Leicester, Leicester, UK

The influence of the autonomic nervous systems (ANS) on dynamic cerebral autoregulation was studied by measuring both middle cerebral artery blood flow (CBFV) via transcranial Doppler ultrasonography and non-invasive arterial blood pressure (ABP) in 53 normal subjects (mean age 66.6 years, range 39-80) at rest and during manoeuvres designed to produce a sudden dynamic change in ABP with simultaneous stimulation of the sympathetic nervous system, (Valsalva manoeuvre, cold pressor test, release of isometric hand grip, thigh cuff release, and lower body negative pressure). The dynamic CBFV response was described using Tiecks model (ARI index) and the moving-average impulse and step responses. Impulse responses were similar for the right and left hemispheres. Their temporal pattern was not influenced by BP manoeuvre, and was similar to the results for spontaneous ABP transients (positive or negative). ARI values were also independent of the manoeuvre (4.4 ± 2.0, N=756 recordings). The amplitude of the impulse and step responses, however, were significantly affected by the manoeuvre used and were highly correlated with the resistance-area product before the sudden change in ABP (r = -0.96, p< 0.0001). These results suggest that the amplitude of the CBFV step response is sensitive to the point of operation of the instantaneous ABP-CBFV relationship that can be altered by different manoeuvres. The sympathetic nervous system activation resulting from different dynamic ABP changes is not reflected by the CBFV dynamic autoregulatory responses within the physiological range of ABP.

111

DYNAMIC CEREBRAL AUTOREGULATION: TRANSFER FUNCTION PHASE AND RESPONSE TO VALSALVA MANEUVERS IN PATIENTS WITH CAROTID ARTERY STENOSIS

M. Reinhard, A. Hetzel, M. Lauk*, and C.H. Lücking
Department of Neurology and Clinical Neurophysiology, University Clinics of Freiburg, Germany
*Center for Data Analysis and Modeling, University of Freiburg, Germany

Background and purpose: Evaluation of dynamic cerebral autoregulation might become a promising, physiologically more appropriate diagnostic tool in assessment of cerebral hemodynamic impairment in patients with carotid artery stenosis than CO_2-reactivity testing. However, little has been published yet on possible clinical application of such tests and knowledge about inter-method agreement is rare. For this reason, two simple non-invasive methods (phase shift during deep breathing and response to Valsalva maneuvers (VM)) were applied and compared to each other and to CO_2-reactivity.

Methods: Nineteen patients with tight carotid artery stenosis and seventeen age-matched controls were examined using transcranial Doppler sonography. Phase shift was determined by cross-spectral analysis, responses to Valsalva maneuvers were graded by the formerly-introduced ASI (autoregulation slope index) and the new VTI (Valsalva time index), which is based solely on time course latencies of cerebral blood flow velocity (CBFV) and blood pressure (ABP).

Results: Phase shift and autoregulatory indices were significantly reduced ipsilateral to the affected side compared to controls ($p<0.0001$) or contralateral sides (from $p=0.0011$ to $p=0.0001$). Correlation with CO_2-reactivity showed significant results when pooling values of controls and patients (r from 0.54 to 0.78; $P<0.001$). However, correlations except for the VTI ($r=-0.65$; $P=0.002$) were not significant considering only the affected side in patients. Correlation of pooled values between phase shift and VM-derived indices was significant (VTI $r=-0.62$; $P<0.001$; ASI $r=0.49$; $P<0.001$), within patients only when comparing side-to-side differences (VTI $r=-0.58$; $P=0.009$; ASI $r=0.52$; $P=0.023$).

Conclusions: Detection of impaired cerebral autoregulation is possible both by deep breathing and VM. However, inter-method agreement concerning the extent of impairment is only acceptable for intraindividual side-to-side differences. The presented results suggest that absolute values of one autoregulation testing method alone or CO_2-reactivity alone might fail to detect impairment in cerebral hemodynamics. Thus CO_2-reactivity and various dynamic cerebral autoregulation tests should be combined for comprehensive assessment of the cerebral hemodynamic functional status in patients with carotid artery stenosis.

112

PARADOX METABOLICALLY INDUCED CHANGES IN REGIONAL CEREBRAL BLOOD FLOW IN PATIENTS WITH SEVERE AXONAL HEAD INJURY AND PRESERVED CEREBRAL AUTOREGULATION

M. Rosenkranz, V.U. Becker, A. Thie*. Dept. of Neurology, University of Hamburg, Germany.*Dept. of Neurology, Gen. Hospital Itzehoe, Germany.

Objective: Cerebral autoregulation (AR) is suggested to be regulated by the same local metabolic mechanisms as flow-metabolism coupling (vasoneuronal coupling). By assessment of metabolically induced cerebral blood flow velocity changes, transcranial Doppler (TCD) offers the opportunity to evaluate vasoneuronal coupling in patients with severe axonal head injury (HI) and preserved AR.

Methods: Within 48h after admission we performed simultaneous TCD recordings from both MCA during focal transcranial magnetic stimulation (TMS) of the right sensorimotor cortex in 13 patients with axonal HI and intact AR. Stimulation energy was 80-100% of maximum output. Non of the subjects had raised intracranial pressure (intraparenchymal pressure probes). Fentanyl and midazolam was administered intravenously to all patients. Using average techniques, mean MCA flow velocities and instantaneous blood pressure traces were assessed.

Results: Following TMS, no potentials in corresponding muscles could be detected. There was a bilateral marked drop in MCA flow velocity in all patients. The decrease was deeper on the left compared to the right side (p<0.05). Flow velocity was restored within 25s in all subjects. There were no side-to-side differences in temporal flow parameters (onset to beginning of flow drop, t_{50}, time to peak (ttp)). Averaged blood pressure traces did not show significant alterations during recordings.

hemisphere	drop [%]	onset [s]	t_{50} [s]	ttp [s]
stimulated (right)	-9.6±2.4	2.7±1.8	4.2±2.2	6.8±2.9
nonstimulated (left)	-10.7±2.1	2.7±1.8	4.1±2.2	6.7±2.9
Wilcoxon-test	p<0.05	n.s.	n.s.	n.s.

Conclusion: In patients with axonal HI, TMS induces steep blood pressure independent short term decreases of cerebral blood flow (CBF) in both hemispheres. Since excitatory and inhibitory neurotransmission is associated with increases and decreases in CBF, respectively, our findings suggest that in axonal HI, excitability of excitatory neurons might be disturbed, while that of inhibitory systems is preserved. The TMS-induced drop in CBF might be due to prevailing activation of local inhibitory mechanisms with subsequent reduction of excitatory synaptic activity and metabolic demand, which is compatible with at least partly intact flow-metabolism coupling.

113

LINEAR COUPLING BETWEEN CEREBRAL AND SYSTEMIC HEMODYNAMICS IN PATIENTS UNDERGOING HEART TRANSPLANTATION - A PROSPECTIVE TRANSCRANIAL DOPPLER SONOGRAPHY STUDY

M. Schneider[1], D.G. Nabavi[2], C. Schmid[1], S. Christiansen[1], S. Kerber[3], D.W. Droste[2], H.H. Scheld[1]. Departments of Cardiothoracic & Vascular Surgery[1], Neurology[2], and Cardiology[3], University of Münster, Germany.

Background and Purpose: Heart transplantation (HTX) is an established treatment for patients with terminal heart disease but appropriate patient selection and postoperative monitoring is still a matter of debate. This prospective study was undertaken to evaluate whether transcranial Doppler sonography (TCD) could serve as an additional prognostic parameter for HTX.

Methods: TCD was performed before HTX (n=63), three days (n=38), and six months (n=24) after HTX. In 10 patients, vasomotor reserve capacity (VMRC) was assessed using azetazolamide (1g i.v.) before HTX and 6 months after HTX. TCD findings were correlated to NYHA stage, clinical course, and to hemodynamic results as obtained by repeated right heart catheterizations.

Results: In two patients, intracerebral hemorrhage occurred 3 and 5 days after HTX during mild arterial hypertension. Mean TCD blood flow velocities significantly increased from pre-HTX examination (49.5±12.6 cm/s [mean±SD]) to early post-HTX (65.7±15.8 cm/s; p< 0.001), followed by slight reduction at late post-HTX exam (56.7±15.9 cm/s, p= 0.03). VMRC strongly increased from 54.3 ± 16.6 % (pre-HTX) to 86.1%±16.8 (post-HTX; p=0.007). TCD values before and early after HTX were in parallel to the course of mean arterial blood pressure and cardiac output.

Conclusions: In patients with end-stage heart disease, cerebral autoregulation is significantly disturbed before and early after HTX with linear coupling between cerebral and systemic hemodynamics. This linear relationship may contribute to the manifestation of peri-procedural brain hemorrhages and other cerebrovascular diseases.

114

TCD-MONITORING IN PATIENTS WITH PITUITARY APOPLEXY

V.B.Semenyutin, Y.I.Vaynshenker, V.F.Melkishev, V.V.Alexeev

Russian Polenov Neurosurgical Institute, St.Petersburg, Russia

Background: Pathogenesis of the pituitary apoplexy (PA) is not well-known. Taking into consideration pronounced hypothalamo-hypophyseal disfunction, it was supposed that development of vasospasm (VS) and intracranial hypertension (ICH) takes place in these patients during PA. To prove this suggestion blood flow velocity (BFV) monitoring was performed after PA in the major arteries at the brain base in different PA forms.

Material and Method: We examined 23 patients with pituitary adenomas of different sizes and histological types. Pronounced symptomatic PA was in 12 cases, and mild or asymptomatic in 11, conformed with CT and MRI. 11 patients had tumors with hemorrhagic content, including 2 subarachnoid, 12 - cystic tumors. TCD-monitoring was performed using the Multi Dop X system (DWL, Germany).

Results: VS and/or ICH were revealed in 19 (82.6%) cases. ICH sings were revealed in the first hours after PA. VS increased and reached maximum on the 5-7th day. Only 2 of 19 patients had VS without ICH signs. In one case in siphon ICA (BFV was 106 cm/s, pulsatility index (PI) - 0.65, Lindegaard's index (LI) - 3.1), in the other - in MCA (BFV was 82 cm/s, PI - 0.62, LI - 3.5). 8 patients had VS accompanied with ICH: BFV in siphon ICA - 140.0±23.6 cm/s, in MCA -129.0±23.0 cm/s, in ACA - 129.8±32.5 cm/s, PI - 1.13±0.10, 1.09±0.15, 1.12±0.18, respectively. 9 patient had evidently ICH without VS: BFV in siphon ICA - 44.5±10.1 cm/s, in MCA - 56.5±9.1 cm/s, in ACA - 48.2±17.8 cm/s, PI - 1.29±0.21, 1.15±0.17, 1.12±0.13, respectively.

Conclusion: PA is accompanied with VS of basal brain arteries and/or ICH. One should consider this fact to treat pituitary adenomas with hemorrhagic and/or cystic content.

115

NON-INVASIVE ASSESSMENT OF ICP DYNAMICS DURING PRESERVED AND DISTURBED AUTOREGULATION

B. Schmidt, M. Czosnyka*, J. Schwarze, J. Klingelhöfer

Dept. of Neurology, Chemnitz Medical Center, Chemnitz, Germany

* Academic Neurosurgical Unit, Addenbrooke's Hospital, Cambridge, UK

Background and Purpose. The autoregulatory state strongly affects cerebral hemodynamics, particularly the interdependencies between flow velocity (FV) in cerebral arteries, ABP and ICP. Autoregulatory reserve may be assessed by correlation coefficients between FV and CPP (Mx) as well as ABP and ICP (PRx). The coefficients Mx and PRx, both introduced by Czosnyka et al. (*Stroke.1996;27:1829-1834*), indicate impaired autoregulation, if positive, and preserved autoregulation, if negative. A recently developed mathematical model estimated a continuous ICP curve from analysis of FV in MCA and ABP signals. Objective of this work was to investigate, whether this ICP simulation would preserve the autoregulatory state. **Methods.** The ICP simulation was split into two versions suitable for traumatic brain injured patients either with disturbed or intact autoregulation. These versions were tested on groups of 30 patients with preserved (group A; Mx and PRx were -0.56 ± 0.16 and -0.41 ± 0.11) and 45 patients with impaired autoregulation (group B; Mx was +0.58 ± 0.23 and PRx was +0.48 ± 0.25). **Results.** Using simulated ICP (instead of direct measured ICP) for calculation of indices, Mx and PRx were -0.64 ± 0.16 and -0.46 ± 0.2 in group A and +0.5 ± 0.24 and +0.41 ± 0.25 in group B. Signs of Mx were preserved by simulation in both groups, while PRx changed signs in 1 patient in group A and 3 patients in B. These sign invariances apart, correlations between real and simulated indices were low (R<0.4) with exception of Mx in group A (R=0.69, P<0.001). Mean error between measured and simulated ICP was 5.5 ± 4.9 mmHg in group A and 7.1 ± 5.6 mmHg in group B. **Conclusion.** The sign invariance of PRx and Mx under simulation indicated corresponding autoregulatory reserves in real and simulated data, not affected by mostly weak correlations between autoregulation indices. The results showed that ICP simulation was able to assess the autoregulation specific ICP dynamics and therefore preserved the autoregulatory states with good reliability. After choosing the correct type of ICP simulation, e.g. by clinical autoregulation tests, trends of ICP could be assessed accurately in a non-invasive manner.

116

A SIMPLE PARAMETRIC FILTER TECHNIQUE FOR QUANTIFYING AUTOREGULATION USING SPONTANEOUS VARIATIONS IN BLOOD PRESSURE

D. M. Simpson*, R. B. Panerai*, A. R. Naylor**, D. H. Evans*

Divisions of Medical Physics* and Surgery**, Faculty of Medicine, University of Leicester, Leicester, LE1 5WW, UK. E-mail: DMS18@LE.AC.UK

Techniques to test cerebral blood flow (CBF) autoregulation often involve manipulation of arterial blood pressure (ABP) which is inconvenient or even dangerous in vulnerable patient groups. The analysis of the interrelation between CBF and ABP during spontaneous variability has been proposed as a simpler means of detecting autoregulation. The expected high-pass filter relationship has been consistently observed, and phase, gain and impulse responses have shown encouraging results. We propose a parametric approach to this problem, using a first order finite-impulse response filter - the simplest possible filter to give a high-pass response. Filter coefficients were estimated from ABP and CBF velocity (CBFV from trancranial Doppler ultrasound) of 60 patients with stenosis (or occlusion) of the carotid arteries. Data were collected during the inspiration of ambient air (normocapnia - NC1), a 5% CO2 / air mixture (hypercapnia - HC) and finally return to ambient air (normocapnia - NC2). Each stage lasted for approximately 2 minutes. Equivalent data were collected in 15 normal subjects. The cerebrovascular reactivity (CVR - % increase in CBFV per unit change in end-tidal pCO2) was calculated. The filters consistently showed high-pass characteristics, which were significantly reduced during HC in the normal subjects ($p<0.002$) and lower in patients than the normals ($p<0.005$). Highly significant correlation between CVR and the filter parameters ($r>0.45$, $p<0.001$) gives further evidence that the filter reflects autoregulation. Large intra- and inter-individual scatter of results however remains the major problem.

117

Reduction of Vasomotor Reactivity is related to the Severity of Cerebral Microangiopathy

Christoph Terborg[1], Felix Gora[1], Cornelius Weiller[2], Joachim Röther[2]
Departments of Neurology, Friedrich – Schiller University of Jena[1], and University Hospital Eppendorf, Hamburg[2], Germany

The aim of our study was to determine whether near-infrared spectroscopy (NIRS) can detect a reduced VMR in patients with microangiopathy, whether NIRS-reactivities correlate with VMR assessed by transcranial Doppler sonography (TCD), and whether different extent of microangiopathy on CT or MRI can be distinguished by both noninvasive techniques.

We compared VMR of 46 patients with cerebral microangiopathy with 13 age-matched controls. Patients were classified using the Erkinjuntti-scale. We monitored cerebral blood flow velocity (CBFV) in both middle cerebral arteries by TCD, changes in concentration of oxyhemoglobin (HbO_2), deoxyhemoglobin (Hb) and blood volume (HbT) by NIRS, mean arterial blood pressure, and endtidal CO_2 ($EtCO_2$) during normo- and hypercapnia. VMR's were calculated as percentage change of CBFV (NCR), and as absolute change in concentration of HbO_2, Hb, and HbT per 1 % increase in $EtCO_2$ (CR-HbO_2, CR-Hb, CR-HbT).

NCR and NIRS-reactivities were significantly reduced in patients with cerebral microangiopathy. CR-HbO_2 and CR-Hb showed a close correlation with NCR, and NCR and NIRS-reactivities were related to the severity of cerebral microangiopathy according to the Erkinjuntti-scale. Validity of NCR and NIRS-reactivities were similar.

VMR is reduced in patients with cerebral microangiopathy and can be noninvasively assessed in basal arteries (TCD) and brain parenchyma (NIRS). Reduction of CO_2-induced VMR as measured by NIRS and TCD may indicate the severity of microangiopathy.

118

TRANSCRANIAL DOPPLER SONOGRAPHY MONITORING OF CEREBRAL ORTHOSTATIC AUTOREGULATION IN ORTHOSTATIC INTOLERANCE: EFFECTS OF GRAVITY AND PERIPHERAL MUSCLE PUMP

E. Titianova[1], I. Velcheva[1], J. Nader[2]
[1]Department of Neurology, Sofia, Bulgaria, [2]National Institute of Neurology and Neurosurgery, Mexico City, Mexico

The study aimed to evaluate the orthostatic adjustment of cerebral hemodynamics in patients with orthostatic intolerance (OI) and to assess the effects of gravity and peripheral muscle pump on its appearance.

Hemodynamic changes associated with orthostatic challenge were studied in 20 healthy volunteers and 40 patients with OI. A passive 70° tilt of the upper part of the body followed by a passive 90° whole body tilting and an active orthostatic stand-up were applied. Mean blood pressure (MBP), heart rate, and mean blood flow velocity of both middle cerebral arteries (monitored by transcranial Doppler sonography) were determined after 10 minutes rest and after 1, 5 and 10 minutes of each orthostatic position.

The pattern of orthostatic adjustment of the cerebral and the common hemodynamics depended on the topic of the lesion and the type ("passive or active") of orthostatic challenge. Gravity forces and peripheral muscle pump influenced mainly the efficacy of the compensatory antigravity mechanisms. In patients with postural tachicardia syndrome a paradoxical cerebral vasoconstriction occurred. In cases with pure autonomic failure the cerebral autoregulation seemed to be preserved if the MBP was maintained within the limit for brain autoregulation. During the induced neurally mediated syncope the selective loss of diastolic blood flow and the increase in pulsatility index were typically observed. The clinical impact of these findings in respect to therapeutic and rehabilitation strategies is discussed.

119

TRANSCRANIAL DOPPLER MONITORING DURING PHYSICAL EXERCISE IN PATIENTS WITH STROKE RISK FACTORS

A.Valikovics, T.Magyar, *I.Czuriga, L.Csiba.
Departments of Neurology and *Cardiology, Health Sience Center, University of Debrecen, H-4012 Debrecen, Hungary.

Background: Dilatory ability of resistance arterioles in patients with major cardiovascular risk factors is impaired. Previously we examined cerebral hemodynamics in hypertensives by TCD monitoring during ergometer cycling. In this study we compared changes of hemodynamic parameters during exercise in patients with one (hypertension) and two (hypertension + hypercholestherinemia) stroke risk factors.

Subjects and methods: 30 hypertensive patients (mean age 42,3±5,3 years) were investigated by TCD during ergometer cycling. 17 patients suffered isolated hypertension (HT) and 13 patients had also hypercholesterinemia (HT+HC). Blood pressure, heart rate, end-tidal CO_2 (Capnogard capnograph), and MCA mean blood flow velocity (Multidop X DWL) were continously monitored during ergometer cycling according to the WHO protocol. ANOVA-test were used for the statistical analysis.

Results: There were no statistically significant differences between HT and HT+HC patients during physical exercise in duration of loading (4,8±2,6 and 4,0±2,8 min; mean±SD), changes of end-tidal CO_2 (20,6±9,8% and 18,8±6,5%) blood pressure (26,2±9,6 and 29,3±10,0%) and changes of mean velocity in MCA (26,3±12,5 and 24,9±9,7%). The ratio of $dMV/etCO_2$ did not differ between the two groups.

Conclusions: However, previously decreased mean velocity changes and $dMV/etCO_2$ ratio were showed in hypertensive patients compared with healthy volunteers during ergometer cycling, we can not find differences in these parameters between the patients with one and with two risk factors.

120

TRANSCRANIAL DOPPLER SONOGRAPHY MONITORING OF VASOMOTOR REACTIVITY OF MIDDLE CEREBRAL ARTERIES IN PATIENTS WITH CEREBROVASCULAR DISEASES

I. Velcheva, E. Titianova, D. Alexandrova, P. Damianov
Department of Neurology - Sofia, Bulgaria

The study aimed to evaluate the CO_2 vasomotor reactivity of both middle cerebral arteries (MCA) under different ventilation conditions in patients with risk factors for cerebrovascular disease (CVD), TIAs and chronic cerebral infarctions using transcranial Doppler sonography (TCD).

TCD monitoring (Multi Dop X4-DWL, Germany) of the blood flow velocity of both MCA arteries during normo-ventilation, hypoventilation and hyperventilation (for at least 30 s) was performed in 28 patients who survived cerebral infarctions in the MCA territory with presence of a residual neurological deficit, 8 patients with TIAs, 33 subjects with risk factors for CVD, and 10 healthy controls. The Vasomotor Reactivity Index (VMRI) of MCA during normo-/hypoventilation and normo-/hyperventilation was calculated automatically as percentage change in velocity. Total VMRI and Vasomotor Range (VMR) were also estimated.

The total VMRI and VMR of MCA were almost symmetrical in the controls. In all patients the mechanism of vasodilatation during hypoventilation was insufficient. Its impairment was more expressed in the cases with a chronic stroke on the infarction side. The vasomotor range was slightly restricted with a vasoconstriction predominating in its structure.

In conclusion, patients with risk factors for CVD, TIAs or chronic cerebral infarctions had a disturbed CO_2 vasomotor reactivity of MCA, their mechanism of cerebral vasodilatation during hypoventilation was insufficient or missing. Therefore, the vasomotor range of cerebral circulation depended more or less on its ability for vasoconstriction during hypocapnia. The clinical importance of these findings needs to be elucidated.

121

STUDY OF BLOOD PRESSURE AND CEREBRAL BLOOD FLOW VELOCITY VARIABILITY IN HYPERTENSIVE PATIENTS AND NORMAL CONTROLS

WJ Wong, HH Hu, TBJ Kuo, WY Sheng, CM Chern, OY Luk
Section of Neurovascular Disease, Neurological Institute, Veterans General Hospital, Taipei, Taiwan

Backgrounds: It is well known that transcranial Doppler monitoring is one of the most reliable and non-invasive technique to evaluate the cerebral artery reserve. The purpose of the study is to using the application of TCD monitoring for assessment of cerebral autoregulation in patients with hypertension and normal controls.
Methods and Results: We conducted normal adults(45 cases) and hypertensive patients(28 cases) for bilateral middle cerebral artery flow velocity (MCAFV) TCD and blood pressure (BP) beat to beat monitoring. 5% CO_2 inhalation was given after a 5 minutes baseline monitoring which spectral and transfer function analyses of MCAFV and BP were performed by fast Fourier transform. There was no significant difference in mean age, sex and other vascular risk factors(DM, smoking, alcohol taking) between the two groups. The results showed that bilateral mean MCAFV were higher in hypertensive group(73.6±24.2 vs 55.4±19, P=0.005) but there was no significant difference in CO_2 reactivity between the two groups. The frequency domain analysis of MCAFV and BP showed lower MCAFV and BP variability of very low frequency in hypertensive patients than normal controls(P=0.007 and P=0.020) but no difference in low frequency and high frequency.
Conclusions: The method of frequency domain analysis of cerebral blood flow velocity and blood pressure had some different results in comparison with CO_2 reactivity test in this study. It needs further study for clarifying the clinical significant of this phenomenon.

122

Transcranial Doppler Investigation After Carotid Surgery

H. Zachrisson, J. Holm, E. Mattson, R. Volkmann.
Departments of Clinical Physiology and Surgery, Sahlgrenska University Hospital, Göteborg, Sweden

Introduction By Transcranial Doppler (TCD) it is possible to measure blood flow velocities in the circle of Willis. In this study TCD was performed the days after carotid thrombendarterectomy (CEA) in order to describe the cerebral hemodynamics after normalisation of the blood flow.

Methods A group of patients with neurological symptoms were referred to postoperative TCD investigation after CEA (S-group, n=6). In addition, consecutive patients without neurological complications (C-group, n=35) were investigated by TCD. The S-group included stroke due to hyperperfusion (n=1), thrombemboli/TIA (3 patients), vertebrobasilar symptoms (n=1) and Horners syndrome (n=1).

Results In most of the patients in the S-group marked or medium increased flow velocities were seen in the anterior part of the circle of Willis. A subgroup in the C-group was identified with high blood pressure and/or headache after operation (n=16). Most of the latter patients showed medium flow velocity increase bilaterally in the anterior part of circle of Willis. Marked flow velocities were seen bilaterally in two of these patients without any symptoms but a high blood pressure postoperatively. Another patient had marked ipsilateral flow velocities at the day when the patient was planned to leave the hospital. The rest of the C-group (n=19) had minor or moderate flow velocity increase in the anterior part of circle of Willis. Most patients had normalised flow velocities in the circle of Willis three months after CEA.

Conclusions After carotid surgery, flow velocity increase is often seen bilaterally in the anterior part of circle of Willis. This can be due to dysfunction of the cerebral autoregulation, baroreceptor dysfunction or vasospasm.

123

TCD FLOW PATTERN IN A NON-INVASIVE MODEL OF INTRACRANIAL PRESSURE

S. Zieroth, M. Stoll
SHG-Kliniken, Dept. of Neurology, D-66663 Merzig, Germany
Hospital for Neurology, D-83043 Bad Aibling, Germany

Introduction: An increase of pulsatility index (PI) as indicator for cerebrovascular resistance in TCD may be a result of hyperventilation (HV) or increased intracranial pressure (ICP). In the first case arteriols constrict in decreased pCO2. The mechanism and site, responsible for the increase of PI in ICP is under discussion. We compared systolic, mean and diastolic flow velocities in TCD during HV and artificially increased ICP in humans to elaborate specific differences in flow pattern. Method: In ten healthy probands (20-35 years) we measured the MCA flow continously bitemporal with TCD. We controlled exspiratory CO2, heart-rate and arterial blood pressure continously. A cervical cuff with controlled pressure was inflated up to 1.3 mmHg per cm circumference of the neck to decrease intracranial venous outflow. Results: After hyperventilation for 25 sec the eCO2 had decreased by 35.89 % ± 18.63 (p< 0.01) and the PI had increased by 0.49 ± 0.28 (p< 0.01). In detail the diastolic flow velocity decreased by 18.09 cm/s ± 8.26 (39.04 % ± 13.87) (p < 0,01) and the systolic flow velocity decreased by 11.38 cm/s ± 7.61 (10.64 % ± 5.67) (p<0.01). There was no significant change of arterial blood pressure after 25 sec. Increasing the ICP by inflating the cuff caused an abrupt reduction of diastolic flow velocity by 9.76 cm/s ± 6.05 (19.89 % ± 11.6) (p<0.05) and hence increase of the PI by 0.26 ± 0.15 (p<0.01) (value after 25 sec.). In contrary to HV there was no significant change of systolic flow velocity (+0,7 ± 5,23 cm/s). After deflation of the cuff the diastolic flow velocity reincreased abruptly to former values. Conclusion: Increasing the ICP by extracranial outflow obstruction the PI increases only by means of a decrease of the diastolic blood flow velocity. During HV, in contrast, systolic and diastolic flow velocity decrease. These TCD criteria may help in distinction between increased incranial pressure and HV as cause for increased PI. The used model is on principle suitable for studies on increased ICP.

124

CEREBROVASCULAR REACTIVITY TO L-ARGININE IN STROKE PATIENTS

Žvan B, Zaletel M, Pogačnik T
University Medical Centre, Dept. of Neurology, Ljubljana, Slovenia.

Objectives: Post-ischemic hypoperfusion may play a significant role in reperfusion injury. The endothelium-dependent vasodilatation should be impaired during hypoperfusion. L-arginine (L-A), a precursor of nitric oxide (NO), is able to elicit endothelium-dependent vasodilatation. To determine the function of the cerebral vascular endothelial function in early stage after ischemic stroke, we studied cerebrovascular reactivity to L-A with TCD.
Methods: The study group consisted of 15 patients, aged 57.6±9.8 years, with the middle cerebral artery syndrome. They were investigated on days 7 to 10 after ischemic stroke. The control group consisted of 15 healthy volunteers, aged 58±10.7 years. All subjects received an intravenous infusion of L-A over 20 minutes at a rate 1.5 g/min. The mean arterial velocity (v_m) was measured in the middle cerebral artery using bitemporal monitoring system (MultiDop X4, DWL). At the same time, the mean arterial pressure (MAP) and heart rate (HR) were measured by Finapress. The end-tidal CO_2 (Et-CO_2) was monitored by capnograph. The v_m over five-minute intervals at rest and during the infusion of L-A was determined by using a software TCD8. We also calculated the Pulsatility index (PI).
Results: The v_m significantly increased in both hemispheres (HEM) of both groups (p=0.00). v_m differences between rest and L-A stimulation were lower in the damaged HEM compared to the healthy one (p=0.00), but did not differ between the ischemic HEM and HEM of the healthy group (p>0.05). PI did not change significantly during L-A infusion in both groups (p>0.05). MAP and HR did not change during an infusion (p>0.05). Et-CO_2 changed significantly during L-A stimulation (p=0.05).
Conclusions: Cerebrovascular reactivity to L-A is impaired in patients with recent stroke. It seems, that endothelium dysfunction is important in reperfusion injury.

125

HARMONIC IMAGING OF THE BRAIN USING GREY SCALE AND POWER DOPPLER TECHNOLOGY

Claassen L., Seidel G., Algermissen Ch., Katzer T.
Dept. of Neurology, Medical University of Lübeck, Germany

Objective: Is is unclear which harmonic imaging mode (Power Doppler or grey scale imaging) is superior and which parameter is the most robust for the description of brain perfusion.
Methods: We performed an animal study using Optison™ in three different doses (0.15, 0.3 and 0.6 ml). Intensity vs. heart cycle plots were generated to evaluate the peak increase from baseline (PI) and the area under the curve (AUC).
Results: With harmonic grey scale imaging we observed in the brain parenchyma a homogenous increase in brightness and a significant dose-dependent increase in PI (p=0.03, respectively; n=5). With harmonic Power Doppler the colour signal was inhomogenous, but the increase of PI and AUC showed significance (p=0.03 and 0.01, respectively, n=6).
Conclusion: Due to a more homogenous increase in brightness grey scale imaging may be more suitable displaying brain perfusion. The peak increase seems the most robust parameter describing cerebral perfusion with both imaging modes.

126

Quantification of flow rates using Harmonic Grey Scale Imaging in an In-Vitro-Model

Claassen L./ Seidel G./ Algermissen Ch./ Katzer T.
Dept. of Neurology, Medical University of Lübeck, Germany
E-mail: claassen_l@neuro.mu-luebeck.de

Abstract
Objective: It is unclear if the dye dilution theory and it's related parameters are capable to measure perfusion using harmonic imaging. **Method:** We performed an in-vitro study using Levovist as the ultrasound contrast agent with six different doses (0.1 ml - 3.0 ml) and eight different flow-rates (30 - 100 RPM). We used the HP SONOS 5500 device in connection with the 1.8 / 3.6 MHz harmonic imaging transducer (S4). According to the dye dilution theory we evaluated the time-intensity curve and the influence of dose and flow-rate on the parameters peak increase (PI), area under the curve (AUC) and mean transit time (MTT) using the software of the ultrasound system. **Results:** The AUC and the PI increased only in the dose range between 0.1 and 1.0 ml Levovist. Further increase led to no increase of AUC or PI. Increasing the flow-rate the AUC and the MTT decreased and the PI didn't change. **Conclusion:** Due to analysing artifacts the dye dilution theory is not a useful theoretical model for the analysis of perfusion using harmonic imaging. Explanations for this effect are first the limited dynamic range of the ultrasound system and second the shadowing artifact which prevents further increase of intensity using high contrast concentrations.

127

DOPPLER POWER INCREASES CAUSED BY INDIVIDUAL CONTRAST BUBBLES

KJ Haggag, D Russell, R Brucher. The Dept. of Neurology, The National Hospital, Oslo, Norway and Ulm University of Applied Sciences, Germany.

Objectives: Contrast agents based on gas-filled bubbles have a considerable potential for increasing the diagnostic possibilities of neurosonological examinations. They should, however, meet several criteria; size distribution and safety being of great importance. The aim of this study was therefore to develop a new method which could be used to study the size distribution of contrast bubbles in vitro by enhanced Doppler power measurements.
Material and methods: Albunex contrast bubbles were introduced into a pulsatile loop system containing a circulating blood substitute (S). Maximum Doppler power reflections from individual contrast bubbles were measured at an insonating frequency of 2 MHz. The relative increase in reflected power compared to the blood substitute (contrast/substitute ratio) CSR was calculated for each bubble. The measurements were carried out during different flow types (pulsatile or non-pulsatile), flow rates (40, 60 or 80 cm/sec) and pressures (70 or110 mBar).
Results: The amount of ultrasound power reflection could be accurately measured for single bubbles and we found the following: (i) The calculated CSR values correlated with size distribution measured by other methods. (ii) There was a significant decrease in CSR values with pressure increase (p<0.05). (iii) There was no significant difference in mean CSR when non-pulsatile was compared with pulsatile flow and for the different flow rates. (iii) There was a slight tendency for CSRs to decrease in systole compared to diastole.
Conclusion: This study shows that the size distribution of individual contrast bubbles may be assessed by measuring the reflected power (dB) from each bubble. Pressure increases caused a decrease in reflected power which is probably due to bubble compression. Changes in flow type or flow rate did not significantly influence the bubble size distribution.

128

Echo-Enhanced Transcranial Color Coded Duplexsonography (eeTCCD) versus Digital Subtraction Angiography (DSA)in the Diagnosis of Intracranial Vascular Diseases.

Hahn G., Kunz A., Bourquain H., Gahn G., Reichmann H.
Department of Neurology, University of Technology Dresden, Germany

OBJECTIVE: To assess the diagnostic efficacy of eeTCCD for noninvasive evaluation of the intracranial vasculature in patients with limited acoustical bone windows.
MATERIAL AND METHODS: In this ongoing trial we so far prospectively examined 11 consecutive patients (1 woman, 10 men, mean age 58,3 ± 10,3) with eeTCCD and DSA for assessment of acute cerebrovascular events. We evaluated 9/11 patients for critical symptomatic internal carotid artery obstruction (3 bilateral, 6 unilateral obstruction).
RESULTS:
In all patients eeTCCD visualized the circle of Willis. DSA and eeTCCD showed collateral flow through the anterior communicating artery (Acom) in 4 patients. In 1 out of these 4 patients DSA and eeTCCD showed additional collateral flow through the posterior communicating artery (Pcom). In another one DSA and eeTCCD found collateral flow exclusively through the Pcom. DSA and eeTCCD conclusively showed no collateral flow through the circle of Willis in 4 patients. In another patient both DSA and eeTCCD identified a left parietooccipital arteriovenous malformation. In a 52 year old woman with known intracranial disease eeTCCD suggested a severe stenosis of the MCA (peak systolic velocity 400 cm/s) DSA was primarily read as normal. Second review of the DSA showed a short segment of severe narrowing in the MCA.
CONCLUSION:
In this ongoing study eeTCCD is an accurate methode for evaluation of intracranial vascular disease. eeTCCD provides important physiologically based information. This may alter the anatomically based information of DSA.

129

Normal values of cerebral circulation time measured by echocontrast-enhanced color-coded duplex sonography.

Andreas Kauert, Stephan Schreiber, Karl Max Einhäupl, José Manuel Valdueza
Department of Neurology, University Hospital Charité, Humboldt University Berlin, Germany

Background and Objective:
Several cerebral vascular and degenerative diseases influence the cerebral circulation time (CCT). In the past CCT has been investigated with methods like angiography, scintigraphy, MRI and extracranial Doppler. This study evaluates CCT with echocontrast-enhanced colour-coded duplex sonography in a group of healthy volunteers.
Methods and Results:
CCT is measured after intravenous bolus injection of the echo contrast enhancer Levovist® as the time interval between bolus arrival in the internal carotid artery and internal jugular vein using an evaluation of the increase of power-Doppler intensity. 40 subjects were studied. Normal values and a correlation with age, sex, body weight, body height, blood flow velocity and volume are being presented.
Conclusion: We demonstrate a new approach of measuring a global cerebral circulation time in healthy volunteers by using echocontrast-enhanced colour-coded duplex sonography. The method offers a new option for the employment of echocontrast agents in functional ultrasound.

130

DOPPLERSONOGRAPHIC MEASUREMENT OF CEREBRAL CIRCULATION TIME IN HEALTHY VOLUNTEERS

S.J.Schreiber, U.Franke, E.Staciole, K.M.Einhäupl, J.M.Valdueza, Dept. of Neurology, University Hospital Charité, Berlin, Germany

Background and Objective: Cerebral circulation time (CCT) is the time period the blood needs to perfuse the brain. It can be assessed by measuring changes of Doppler intensity after i.v. bolus injection of a galactose based echo-contrast agent (Levovist®). The study investigates normal values and their correlation to age, sex, heart rate, body surface area, systolic blood pressure, endexpiratory CO_2 and arm-to-brain-time in healthy volunteers of different age.
Method and Results: We measured CCT, defined as the time between contrast bolus arrival in the extracranial internal carotid artery and the internal jugular vein, at the submandibular level. Levovist® bolus injection was given into an antecubital vein. 52 healthy volunteers, (23 males, 29 females) aged between 23 and 69 years and free of relevant atherosclerosis or carotid artery disease were studied. In addition reproducibility studies were performed. CCT was 4.6 to 10.2 seconds (mean ± sd: 6.93 ± 1.217 sec). Multivariant regression analysis showed a significant influence for heart rate, systolic blood pressure, endexpiratory CO_2 and arm-to-brain-time. Under hyperventilation CCT increased by 2.1 to 7.3 seconds (3,8 ± 2,36 sec).
Conclusions: Contrast enhanced Doppler-sonography is a suitable, easy and reliable method to measure cerebral circulation time in healthy volunteers of different age. The obtained values are in good correlation with the previously published circulation times determined by angiography. The study sets a basis for further investigation of CCT in different diseases of the brain.

131

INFLUENCE OF EXTERNAL TISSUE HEMODYNAMICS ON NON-INVASIVE ICP MONITORING

A. Ragauskas, V. Petkus, G. Daubaris, V. Deltuva, A. Matukevicius
University of Technology and Medical University, Kaunas, Lithuania

Objective: The sonographic non-invasive ICP monitoring was investigated in our previous works (1). The objective of this study is to determine the influence that the acoustic parameter dynamics of the external tissue/skull bones make on the long-term ICP monitoring accuracy under the neurosurgical ICU conditions.
Methods: A new non-invasive ICP monitor (VITTAMED) that includes the real-time and *in situ* automatic compensation of the influence of extracranial tissues and skull bones has been created. 15 head-injured coma patients were monitored simultaneously both invasively (CAMINO) and non-invasively (11 males, 4 females, age average 42 years, GCS 3-13) in ICU. The comparative studies were performed for patients in different states of cerebral blood flow autoregulation, when ICP was varying bellow and above the critical level of 20-25mmHg. Also, the breathing-hold and hyperventilation tests and the long term (over 3hrs.) non-invasive ICP monitoring were performed during the investigation.
Results: It has been shown experimentally that the real time and *in situ* compensation of acoustic parameters of extracranial tissues and skull bones allows to reduce the drift of measurement data and to achieve acceptable accuracy of the non-invasive ICP monitor. It also has been shown, that the difference between invasive and non-invasive ICP measurement data during the long term monitoring, breathing-hold and hyperventilation tests did not exceed +/- 2mmHg at any given moment.
Conclusion: The comparative studies of the new non-invasive sonographic ICP monitor (VITTAMED) in neurosurgical ICU have shown that by applying the real time and *in situ* compensation of the influence of the extracranial tissue and skull bones to the measured data it is possible to achieve the uncertainty less than +/- 2mmHg for the long term non-invasive ICP monitoring.

1. Ragauskas A. et al. Cerebrovasc Dis 1999;9 (suppl 2):31 and 46

132

TRANSCRANIAL COLOR-CODED DUPLEX SONOGRAPHY OF THE CAROTID SIPHON

Valaikiene J[1], Schlachetzki F[2], Hoelscher T[2], Bogdahn U[2]
Dep. of Neurology, Universities of Vilnius[1], Lithuania, and Regensburg[2], Germany

Introduction: The carotid siphon has an anatomically variant course and is often difficult to assess. Thus, atherosclerotic lesions in this segment of internal carotid artery (ICA) are sometimes overlooked even in angiograms. Yet, they may lead to different therapeutic strategies in the surgical or interventional management of these patients. Transcranial color-coded duplex sonography (TCCS) is a reliable method in the assessment of the basal cerebral arteries and, in contrast to conventional transcranial Doppler, allows for direct visualisation of the cerebral arteries. In this study we investigated the feasibility of TCCS in the evaluation of the carotid siphon segments C1-2 as well as C4-5 with the emphasis on: 1) the establishment of blood flow velocities (peak systolic/end diastolic/mean flow), 2) the pulsatility and resistance indices at 2 defined points within the intracranial portion of ICA (C1-2 and C4-5 segments), 3) the establishment the siphon/MCA ratio and 4) the creation of a standardised protocol to the examine carotid siphon. **Material and methods:** 32 healthy volunteers (mean age 37,8±11,5: 20 women,12 men) without vascular risk factors and history of cerebrovascular disease were examined with TCCS. All subjects had an adequate ultrasonic window and no pathological findings in extracranial cerebral arteries. **Results:** Identification rate for C1-2 segments was 100% (64/64), for C4-5 segment 98% (63/64) employing a standardised approach with two coronal image planes. The maximal systolic velocity for C1-2 and C4-5 was 65±27/54±20 (mean value ± standard deviation), end diastolic-27±11/22±9, mean velocity - 43±18/33±13, pulsatility index-0.94±0.2/1.01±0.2 and resistance index- 0.59±0.07/0.60±0.08. The calculated carotid siphon indices (C1-2/M1 and C4-5/M1) were 0.6±0.2 and 0.5±0.2. **Conclusions:** Our study indicates that TCCS is a reliable tool for carotid siphon evaluation in the segments C1-2 and C4-5, whereas the C3 segment identification remains problematic. The most robust parameters seem to be the resistance and pulsatility indices. Further studies with/without intra- as well as extracranial stenotic leasons have to be persuaded in comparison with the "gold standard" angiography

133

How Reliable is MRA at Predicting Intracranial Stenosis?

Thomas H. Alexander RVT, Robert Burton MD, Lester Collins MD, Preston Harrison MD, Wayne Hostetler MD, Richard Ulrich MD. Southwestern Cerebral Circulatory Dynamics, East Texas Neurology Clinic, East Texas Neurological Institute. Tyler, Texas USA

OBJECTIVE - To investigate the accuracy of MRA (magnetic resonance angiography) in the diagnosis of intracranial artery stenosis.

METHODS - When comparing transcranial Doppler (TCD) studies to MRA and conventional angiography, the test sensitivity (percentage of false negatives) was markedly lower (59% to 80%) versus MRA than with conventional angiography. The diagnostic studies done on two patients seen within a 14 day period with MRA diagnosed right internal carotid stenosis highlight this statistical discrepency.

CONCLUSIONS - MRA should not be the sole diagnostic tool for intracranial artery stenosis, however, when complemented with TCD, conventional angiography can be obviated in many instances.

134

What is an Importance of Transcranial Color-Code Sonography for a Selection of Patients Treated by rt-PA ?

Michal Bar M.D.
Department of Neurology
Teaching Hospital Ostrava-Poruba
Czech Republic

The rules of treatment patients with acute stroke were set on basis of NINDS study. This study was published on 1995 . The conclusion of study was clear : despite an increased incidence of symptomatic intracerebral hemorrhage , treatment with intravenous t-PA within three hours of the onset of ischemic stroke improved clinical outcome at three months Basic inclusion and exclusion criterias were defined. During next period some probles were appeared:

- setting the time from onset of stroke to treatment of stroke with rt-PA
- CT findigs- what brings to us
- which subtype of stroke is eligible to treatment
- decision between intravenous and intraarterial application
- How to examine the patients before the treatment

Author analyzes two cases of patients treated with rt-PA during february 2000. Both patients were examined by CT and TCCS. He sumarizes resultes of treatment and he marks out an importance of TCCS examination for selection of patients eligible for intravenous application of rt-PA.

135

The Doppler characteristics of young patients with stroke

Vanja Bašić, Nikica Thaller, Vesna Đermanović, Vida Demarin

Department of Neurology, University Hospital, "Sestre milosrdnice", Zagreb, Croatia

The purpose of this study was to evaluate the Dopller characteristics of young patients with stroke.

Sixty-two cases of ischemic stroke in Craoatian subjects aged 26 to 49 years are reviewed.We investigated the Color Doppler Flow Imaging (CDFI) and TCD in every patient with stroke. The stroke was diagnosed clinically by neurologist and by CT.

The results showed that fifty of them had large infarctions, as diagnosed by CT scan. Non invasive carotid flow studies revealed a large number of patients with occlusive cerebrovascular disease. In women's group of patients we found that CDFI was normal in 13 cases (52%), tortuotic artery was found in 6 cases (24%), stenosis of internal carotid artery 50-60% in 4 cases (16%), and subtotal stenosis of the signs of vertebral artery hypoperfusion in 1 case (4%). TCD was normal in 18 cases (72%), generalised hypoperfusion in 4 cases (16&) and the signs of vertebral artery hypoperfusion in 3 cases (12%). Between men CDFI was normal in 25 cases (68%), in 7 cases we found occlusion of internal carotid artery (19%), subtotal stenosis of internal carotid artery in 2 cases (55), and in one case we found occlusion of both internal carotid arteries + subtotal stenosis of right external carotid artery + stenosis of left internal carotid artery 90%. TCD was normal in 27 cases (73%), in 7 cases we found hypoperfusion (19%), stenosis of medial cerebral artery in two cases (5%) and in one case we found the signs of vertebral artery hypoperfusion.

Non-invasive carotid flow studies revealed a large number of patients with occlusive cerebrovascular disease.

136

The evaluation of the patients with ischemia in vertebrobasilar territory

Vanja Bašić, Nikica Thaller, Arijana Lovrenčić-Huzjan, Vida Demarin

Department of Neurology, University Hospital "Sestre milosrdnice", Zagreb, Croatia

In order to evaluate pathologic findings in vertebral arteries we studied 80 consecutive inpatients with the symptomatology of vertebrobasilar ischemic disease by means of color Doppler and Transcranial Doppler (CDFI).

The vertebrobasilar ischemic disease in the patients was characterised by abrupt duration and polymorphism of symptoms. In the diagnosis, radiological examination of cervical vertebrae column, Doppler sonography, brain computerised tomography (CT) and electrocardiography were used. Risk factors for ischemic disease were also analysed. CDFI of carotid and vertebral arteries was performed by Acuson 128 XP.

There were 74% female and 26% male patients, age range 23-85. The most frequent subjective symptoms were:dizziness, nausea, general weakens anf falling in one direction.

More than 40% of patients had hypertension. Diabetes mellitus was found in one case. The lipidogram was abnormal in 17% of patients. ECG was abnormal 15%.

CT findings were: normal findings (69%), cortical atrophy (19%), lacunae (4%) and 2% had ischemic changes. CDFI revealed vertebral artery occlusion (10%), and hypoplastic vertebral artery (26%). The rest of patients had the signs of diminished perfusion, and some of them had a normal perfusion.

CDFI of vertebral arteries is important method in estimation of its pathology (hypoplasia, occlusion).

137

The frequency of not-significant extracranial stenosis of carotid arteries in symptomatic patients

Vanja Bašić, Nikica Thaller, Arijana Lovrenčić-Huzjan, Nevenka Blažić-Čop, Vida Demarin

Department of Neurology, University hospital "Sestre milosrdnice", Zagreb, Croatia

The study included 140 stroke patients with mild and moderate extracranial carotid artery stenosis diagnosed by means of color Doppler flow imaging (CDFI). Brain computed tomography (CT) scanning was done for each patient and risk factors were analyzed. There were twelve (31%) female and twenty-six (69%) male patients, with the mean age 67.8 years. Risk factors were: hypertension (84%) and diabetes mellitus (28%). The stenosis of left, right, or both carotid artery was found in 38 patients (27%).

Mild and moderate stenosis of left carotid artery were found in 15 (11%), of right in 9 (6%) and in 14 (10%) patients of both carotid artery. The neurological examination pointed out that in the group of the patients with stenosis of left carotid artery, 46% of patients had left side hemiparesis, 46% had right side hemiparesis, while one patient was dysphatic. The patients with stenosis of right carotid artery had almost the same neurological picture. In the group of the patients who had stenosis of both carotid arteries, 50% had right side hemiparesis, 21% had left side, 21% had dizziness, and 14% had the signs of dementia. In the cases with similar stenosis of both carotid arteries, the neurological deficit of right side was found in 75%. The half of patients with predominant stenosis of left carotid artery, in 50% showed the signs of dementia, 25% had dizziness and paresis of left side was found in 25%, while the patients with predominant stenosis of right carotid artery in 100% had the deficit of right extremities. Brain CT findings showed ischemia of the arterial territory to be the most common sequel of not significant stenosis of one or both carotid artery (42%), followed by multiple lesions in 34%, while the signs of periventricular hypoperfusion were found in 23% of the patients.

The not-significant carotid artery stenosis is often symptomatic more than significant carotid artery stenosis of the opposite side, so we point out the significance of hemodynamic role of the whole circle of Willis.

138

EVALUATION OF BLOOD FLOW VECOCITY AND CEREBROVASCULAR REACTIVITY IN PATIENTS WITH POSTERIOR CIRCULATION INSUFFICIENCY.

Pierzchała K, Kwieciński J, Kapustecki J,.
Department of Neurology Silesian School of Medicine, Zabrze, Poland

Since ischaemic stroke is very widespread, a rapid development of ultrasound diagnostic techniques searching the relationship between cerebral circulation efficiency and pathophysiology of ischaemic lesions is observed. The aim of our study was to evaluate blood flow velocity (BFV)and cerebrovascular reactivity (CVR) of some anterior circulation arteries (MCA) and posterior circulation arteries (PCA, VA)in patients with posterior circulation insufficiency. Material and methods: the study group consisted of 19 patients (13 male, 6 female) of mean age 55±13 yr. Neurological examination, brain CT and TCD were performed in each patients. All patients underwent TCD examination, including evaluation BFV and CVR of both MCA's PCA's and VA's using TC 2020 Pioneer (EME). Control group consisted of 22 healthy volunteers of mean age 59,6±6,3yr. Results: BFV and CVR of MCA, PCA, VA in examined patients were similar compared to controls. CVR of MCA's were non significant different compared to CVR of PCA's and VA's. CVR of posterior circulation arteries in patients with cerebellar syndrome was significantly lower compared to patients with pyramido-cerebellar syndrome. BFV correlated significantly with CVR in VA right and PCA left (r=0,751, r=0,814 respectively). Conclusions: Except CVR impairment, some other additional factors play role in pathogenesis of posterior circulation insufficiency.

139

RECANALIZATION OF ACUTE SYMPTOMATIC OCCLUSIONS OF THE INTERNAL CAROTID ARTERY

S. H. Meves, A. Muhs, J. Federlein, Th. Büttner, Th. Postert
Department of Neurology, St. Josef-Hospital, Ruhr-University, Bochum, Germany

Introduction Spontaneous recanalization of an occluded intracerebral artery is a well described phenomenon. Little is known about the natural course of internal carotid artery (ICA) occlusion and its possible recanalization. The present study was designed to evaluate recanalization rates of the occluded extracranial ICA in acute stroke patients.

Methods 304 patients with an acute ischemia in the territory of the middle cerebral artery were included in this study. All patients had a neurological examination on admission and on discharge. Extracranial and transcranial color-coded sonography was immediately performed after admission and within 7 days. All patients received a cranial computed tomography on admission and within 7 days in order to determine infarct size and localization.

Results 254 patients had no sign of hemodynamic relevant stenosis of the ICA. 21 patients revealed symptomatic high grade ICA stenosis. Of the 30 patients with ICA occlusions, six (20%) patients (5 male, 1 female; age range 57 to 77 years) showed in the control color-coded sonography a recanalization of the ICA. Two patients with embolic occlusion of the ICA due to atrial fibrilliation had the most favourable outcome (64 year old female: ESS-score on admission 32 versus 77 on discharge; 77 year old male: 29 versus 91). There was no residual stenosis in both patients. 4 patients who had ultrasound findings consistent with atherosclerosis in followm up examination (2 high-grade stenosis, 2 with carotid plaques) did not show a remarkable improvement of their ESS-score. Patients with carotid plaques developed complete MCA infarctions, the other 4 patients had partial anterior circulation infarction on follow up CT scan.

Conclusions Recanalization in arteries with a big calibre is not expected. The present study showed that recanalization of the occluded ICA in acute stroke patients is more often than generally presumed. Acute ICA occlusions have been associated with a poor prognosis up to the present. The detection of spontaneous recanalization might help to predict clinical outcome.

140

TRANSIENT ARREST OF CERBRAL BLOOD FLOW IN AN INTRACRANIAL CAROTID ARTERY STENOSIS AS AN INDICATION FOR A MOBILE INTRAVASAL THROMBUS?

C. SAMII, RR. DIEHL, P. BERLIT

Department of Neurology with Clinical Neurophysiology, Alfried-Krupp von Bohlen und Halbach Krankenhaus, Alfried-Krupp-Strasse 21, D-45117 Essen, Germany.

Background: Transcranial color-coded duplex (TCCD) sonography and transcranial Doppler (TCD) monitoring enables assessment of hemodynamic and embolic mechanisms in cerebrovascular disease. We describe a so far unknown hemodynamic phenomenon possibly indicating an intravasal thrombus.
Case description: We report the case of a patient with a transient ischemia in the brain stem territory. Clinically asymptomatic stenosis of left intracranial internal carotid artery (ICA) was detected by means of TCCD. Both TCCD and TCD revealed sudden transient arrest of cerebral blood flow in pre- and poststenotic ICA segments. Hemodynamic parameters assessed by Finapres® were unaffected. Emboli-like signals were detected in poststenotic vessels only.
Conclusions: We assume that in our patient a mobile thrombus in the ICA siphon may have caused the described ultrasound findings due to transient vessel occlusions.

142

Brain Supplying Arteries in Need of Ultrasound Monitoring During and After Neck Radiation ? - A Case Report

JJ Schwarze[1], D Sander[2], J Klingelhöfer[1]
Department of Neurology, Chemnitz Medical Center[1] and Technical University Munich[2], Germany

A 57 year old male was admitted to our service because of mild gait disturbance which he first noticed 10 days prior to admission. The symptoms had not been progressing since then. The patient did not have any cerebrovascular risk factors including prior stroke, TIA or cardiac dieseases. His past medical history was significant only for a lymphoma that was diagnosed 18 months prior to this admission. The lypmphoma had primarily affected lymph nodes in the right neck region, and was surgically removed, and thereafter treated with radiation therapy. A CT-scan that was obtained upon this admission to our service revealed an old infarct in his right cerebellar hemisphere. Although the current CT scan did not show any recent lesions, the old infarct led to believe that cerebrovascular disease may have been a possible underlying cause for the current symptoms, too. Hence, the patient was put on low-dose anticoagulation treatment with heparin. Over the following 8 hours he developed an aphonic voice, severe swallowing problems, mild dyspnea, a persistent singultus, and paresthesia on his right hand and left cheek. Due to the progression of his symptoms the dose of heparin was increased to bring the aPTT to 2.5-fold the initial value.
An MRI obtained soon after the onset of the new symptoms showed in addition to the old cerebellar infarct a recent small lesion in the right half of the medulla oblongata. A Doppler and Duplex examination revealed signs of a proximal occluion of his right vertebral artery while the left vertebral artery and the basilar artery had slightly elevated flow velocities, but otherwise normal signals.
It is postulated that the radiation therapy of the right neck region has led to an occlusion of the posterior inferior cerebellar artery some time ago and, more recently, to a complete occlusion of the right vertebral artery. Possible vascular damage due to radiation therapy is well known for small arteries, much less though, for large arteries, such as the carotid or vertebral arteries. Hence, it is suggested that patients undergoing radiation therapy of the neck region may benefit from monitoring of the brain supplying arteries with ultrasound for some time during and after the treatment.

141

NON-INVASIVE DETECTION OF INTRACRANIAL STENOSES

D.Školoudík, V.Chudoba, D.Václavík, J.Slavík, Č.Majvald
City Hospital Vítkovice, Ostrava, Czech Republic

Transcranial color-coded real-time sonography /TCCS/ and magnetic resonance angiography /MRA/ are new non-invasive techniques for the diagnosis of intracranial vascular stenoses. Over a period of 21 months, the autors identified - using conventional TCCS or contrast-enhanced TCCS /CE-TCCS/ - a total of 130 intracranial vascular stenoses in 43 patients. To improve visualisation of the intracranial arteries, the autors additionaly used, in 28 cases, the echocontrast agent Levovist®. To establish the diagnostic accuracy of TCCS and CE-TCCS, MRA, and angiography, the autors developed their own criteria for the diagnosis and classification of stenoses. CE TCCS was capable of identifying 2.6 times more stenoses than conventional TCCS; the number of stenoses detected by TCCS and CE-TCCS was identical in only 8 cases /28%/. Thirty-two patients /with 90 stenoses identified by ultrasound/ were able to undergo MRA which confirmed 84 stenoses /93%/. In 10 patients with a total of 36 stenoses /detected by ultrasound/, angiography was performed comfirming 35 stenoses /97%/. Ultrasound-based classification of intracranial vascular stenoses by transcranial techniques correlated with the results of MRA in 63 cases /70%/, and those of angiography in 28 cases /78%/. A total of 27 stenoses /in nine patients/ were classified by all three methods /TCCS/CE-TCCS, MRA, angiography/ with complete agreement in stenosis grading in 15 cases /56%/.

143

Abnormal anatomy of vertebrobasilar arteries in patients with dyscirculation in this system.

G.V. Baltgaile, T.N. Timofejeva
Latvian Medical Academy, Riga, Latvia

There are wellknown different kinds of dyscirculation in vertebrobasilar (v-b) arteries system caused by inherent vessels anomalies such as vascular malformations, aneurisms, fibromuscular dysplasia. Another aspect of the question is that the anatomy of intracranial arteries of v-b system is various, and abnormal vessels' branching, confluence, kinking can be found quite often. It's important to recognize whether such vessels' abnormality could be the reason of the disturbance in v-b system.

We are presenting 6 cases of plexiform, dilated, kinked and dysplastic basilar artery (BA) and confluence of vetebral arteries (VA) from 12 analysed cases of different types of anatomical abnormalities of v-b arteries detected by performing TCCD (ATL, HDI 3000 equipment) and confirmed by radiological examinations.

2 children and 4 adult patients had v-b artery syndrome as well as headache and panic attacks.

Pathological changes in blood flow as a high flow velocitie's gradient, flow turbulence with abnormal acoustic phenomena were detected in basilar artery and its branches insonated by transforaminal approach. The dysplasia of basilar artery discovered by using Power imaging regime was accompanied by abnormal musical sounds registered in dopplerogramms. Signs of congestion in basal veins Rozenthal were detected in all cases.

144

Haemodinamical and clinical role of occluded vertebral artery

Vanja Bašić, Nikica Thaller, Arijana Lovrenčić-Huzjan, Vida Demarin

Department of Neurology, University Hospital, "Sestre milosrdnice", Zagreb, Croatia

The incidence of occluded vertebral arteries (VA) in 140 stroke patients treated in Department of neurology in one year period was evaluated. The criteria for extracranial VA occlusion were positive vessel identification, absent flow, presence of collateral flow.

Brain computer tomography (CT), color Doppler of carotid and vertebral arteries were performed in all patients. Risk factors were assessed by lipidogram, blood glucose and presence of hypertension and cardiovascular diseases.

In the group of 140 patients, the occlusion of VA in extracranial part was found in 19 patients (15 males and 4 females). The mean age was 66.8 years.

Risk factors were: pathological lipidogram (36.8 %), hypertension (63%) and diabetes mellitus (26%).

Seven patients with occlusion of one VA, had concommitent significant stenosis of internal carotid artery (three patients had subtotal stenosis of left and one of right ACI, one had 75% stenosis of left ACI, while in one case we found occlusion of left ACI), and the rest of patients had normal carotid arteries.

Brain CT findings showed: ischemia of arterial territory (42%), cortical atrophy (31%) and multiple lesions (26%). No normal brain CT was found.

The present study pointed to the importance of vertebral arteries in patophysiology of stroke, also the frequent findings of occluded VA together with significant stenosis of ACI.

145

AGE DEPENDENT VARIATIONS IN CEREBRAL HEMODYNAMICS AFTER MENTAL STRESS.

S. Castellani*, I. Carobbi**, N. Boni*, C. Zeloni*, V. Corsoni*, S. Fumagalli**, G.F. Gensini*, G. Masotti**

Dipartimento di area critica medica e chrurgica -*Sez. Clinica Medica Generale e Cardiologia; **Sez. Gerontologia Geriatria e Clinica Urologica; University of Florence, Italy

Cerebral blood flow and glucose metabolism in CNS decrease with age. Still undefined is the problem on whether the the ageing process can also induce significant variations in cerebral vascular reactions to cognitive stimuli that can determine an activation of cerebral glucose metabolism. Aim of this study was to investigate the effects of a mental stimulation (Fair culture test) on cerebral hemodynamics in the elderly. 10 young healthy normotensives (age 21 to 31 yrs, mean 24,5), and 10 healthy elderly subjects (age 60 to 69 yrs, mean 64,5) were studied. They were all non-smokers, had a BMI < 27, and were not offspring of diabetic or hypertensive patients. Major psychiatric and neurologic disorders had been ruled out in all subjects before entering the study and all showed a Mini Mental Test score >24. Cerebral hemodynamics was bilaterally investigated with transcranial Doppler (MultiDop x 4 DWL) by measuring the mean velocity in the middle cerebral artery (MCA-Vm) through the temporal windows by two 2 MHz probes. Arterial blood pressure (Finapres) and CO_2 (Datex Normocap CO_2 monitor) were simultaneously recorded. During the whole experiment all subjects were studied in a supine position. After a 10 minute baseline stabilization period, mental stress (Fair Culture test) was administered for 20 minutes to all subjects. The stimulus was followed by a recovery period that lasted until all hemodynamic variables had reverted to baseline. In both groups the stress induced anxiety reaction led to an effective adrenergic stimulation as demonstrated by the significant increase in blood pressure and heart rate. Mean blood pressure increased in the elderly more than in the young during MS (+10.4 % vs. baseline, p<0.03 at peak in the young; +15.1% vs. baseline, p<0,0008 at peak in the elderly). The increase persisted for 10 minutes during the recovery period only in the young, while blood pressure suddenly reverted to baseline soon after MS in the elderly. In the young mean flow velocity significantly increased in the left MCA more than in the right one during the mental stimulation. (+27.8%, p<0.03 in right MCA vs baseline and +34.7 % p< 0,001 in left MCA vs. baseline). The velocities did not significantly change in the elderly. In conclusion, MS leads to significant systemic adrenergic activation in both groups and to significant increases in MCA mean velocities only in the young. This lack of stimulated augmentation in cerebral hemodynamics may indicate that the elderly subjects exhibit a sluggish adaptation to acute increases in metabolic demands imposed by cognitive effort.

146

CEREBRAL HEMODYNAMICS IN VASOVAGAL SYNCOPE

S. Cencetti, A. Rossi, L. Fattorini, A. Montigiani, S. Bacalli, A. Lagi

Department of Internal Medicine 1, Santa Maria Nuova Hospital, Firenze, Italy

Background and Purpose. Cerebral vasoconstriction preceding vasovagal syncope (VVS) has been already described [Grubb BP, *Circulation* 1991]: it has been considered a paradoxical local reaction, because in the rest of the peripheral circulation we can observe a vasodilation [Robinson BJ, *Clin Sci* 1988]. We aimed to assess presence of cerebral vasoconstriction in VVS induced by head-upright tilt (HUT) and to search for its eventual relation with symptoms onset.

Methods. Monitoring of ECG, blood pressure, TCD, breathing and P_{CO2} signals during HUT in 5 young males (mean age 25.8 years) with clinical history of recurrent syncope. Values were averaged over consecutive 20-second boxes. Pulsatility index (PI) was chosen as indirect index of cerebrovascular resistance (CVR). Nonparametric statistics (Mann-Whitney *U* test) were used for paired and unpaired data. Linear regression analysi was performed over CBF velocity and P_{CO2} changes.

Results. All subjects experienced VVS during HUT. Significant increase in respiratory tidal volumes lead to P_{CO2} decrease and to subsequent decrease of mean and diastolic CBF velocities together with PI increase. Significant blood pressure drops occurred 140-180 seconds later. The full-blown vasovagal reaction (bradycardia and hypotension) associated to symptoms of incumbent syncope occurred 180-220 seconds after the CVR increase. Linear regression analysis showed significant relation between P_{CO2} and CBF velocity decreases.

Conclusions. Cerebral vasoconstriction preceding HUT-induced VVS is the physiological consequence of hypocapnia induced by the changes of the respiratory pattern. The delay of symptoms onset (at least 180 seconds) does not suggest that CVR increase is determinant for VVS onset

147

THE CEREBRAL VENOUS HEMODYNAMICS IN PATIENTS WITH UNCOMPLICATED ARTERIAL HYPERTENSION INVESTIGATED BY TRANSCRANIAL COLOR-CODED DUPLEX SONOGRAPHY

A. Chechetkin, Y. Varakin, A. Kouguev, G. Gornostaeva, O. Rebrova

Moscow Institute of Neurology, Russia

Background and purpose. Arterial hypertension (AH) is one of the main risk factors of cerebrovascular diseases. The venous system, as well as the arterial one, is involved in the pathological process in patients with AH. The morphological investigations showed that the veins of the deep brain structures are more volurable. The aim of the study is to assess cerebral blood outflow throughout the deep brain veins.

Material and Methods. We have investigated two groups of patients (male aged 47-65 years). The 1 group included 25 men with normal arterial blood pressure (139/89 mm Hg and lower) and the 2 group included 47 patients with mild to moderate uncomplicated AH. The duration of AH was 5 years or more. The patients with cerebrovascular and cardiopulmanary disease were excluded from the study. The straight sinuses (SS), great cerebral vein (GCV) and basal vein (BV) were insonated. Intracranial vein and SS were studied by "Ultramark-9" (ATL, USA) device equipped with a 2-3 MHz sector scan transducer. The peak systolic (PSV), end-diastolic (PDV) velocities and resistance indices (RI) were determined.

Results. In 1 group PSV in BV was 14,9±3,1 cm/s, in GCV - 19,0±3,8 cm/s, in SS - 26,1±7,3 cm/s; PDV in BV was 11,1±2,5 cm/s, in GCV - 13,8±2,8 cm/s, in SS - 18,0±5,3 cm/s; RI in BV was 0,25±0,04, in GCV - 0,28±0,05, in SS - 0,31±0,04. In 2 group PSV in BV was 12,4±3,3 cm/s, in GCV - 20,4±4,7 cm/s, in SS - 25,4±7,5 cm/s; PDV in BV was 9,0±2,3 cm/s, in GCV - 14,6±3,1 cm/s, in SS - 17,8,0±5,6 cm/s; RI in BV was 0,27±0,04, in GCV - 0,28±0,05, in SS - 0,31±0,04. Statistically significant differences were obtained only for BV. PVS and PVD were lower and RI higher in patient with AH.

Conclusions. There are no significant changes of cerebral venous flow was established in patients with uncomplicated AH, that was showed by statistical analysis including results of values of flow in GCV and SS. However the reduction of outflow in BV show the existence of slight reduction of venous out flow.

148

CAROTID ARTERY ATHEROSCLEROTIC CHANGES IN PATIENTS WITH SYMPTOMATIC CEREBRAL ISCHEMIA

D. Gachechiladze, I. Diasamidze, F. Todua
Institute of Radiology and Interventional Diagnostics/ Tbilisi / Georgia

Purpose: To assess the degree of Carotid artery (CA) stenosis and the structure of atherosclerotic plaques in patients with symptomatic cerebral ischemia.
Matherials and Methods: 130 patients (74 male, 56 female) with focal hemispheric symptoms (64-TIA, 66-Stroke) and sonographically diagnosted ICA stenosis were investigated. MR-Tomography, MR-Angiography and Color-Doppler of exrtacranial vessels was performed.
Results: MRT showed anterior circulation infarction in all stroke patients. In 25(39.1%) TIA patients multiple Lacunar infarctions were diagnosted. Investigation showed increasion of mean CCA Intima-media layer thickening (1.01mm.-TIA, 1.12mm.-Stroke). In 84(64.6%) of cases bilateral CA stenosis was marked. Stroke patients had high frequency of moderate to severe CA stenosis (11\16.7%\-mild, 31\47%\-moderate, 24\36.4%\-severe). TIA patients had a higher frequency of mild to moderate CA stenosis (20\31.3%\-mild, 28\43.8%\-moderate, 16\25%\-severe). Prevalence of potentially unstable ("soft" or "heterogenous") was marked- 38(59.4%)-TIA, 43(65.2%)-stroke.
Conclusion: Stroke patients showes prevalence of high grade CA stenosis. The embolism from unstable plaque may be cause of focal ischemia distal to a symptomatic CA stenosis. Complex use of Color-Doppler and MR-angiography gives all valuable information about extracranial CA hemodinamicaly significant and embologenic stenosis.

149

LASER CAN DETECT MICROEMBOLI : COMPARISON WITH HIGH INTENSITY TRANSIENT SIGNALS BY TCD

Hanzawa K, Sankai Y* , Koguchi H*, Furui E**, Kitamura M, Hayashi J, Naritomi H****, Cardiovasc. Surg., Niigata Univ., *Inst. of Engineer., Tsukuba Univ. ,**Neurology, Kanzawa Univ., *** Cerebrovasc. Div. National Cardiovasc. Center, Japan

Purpose: We attempted to detect microemboli by laser photomotory during left ventricular assist devices (LVAD)
Methods: LVAD was implanted in pigs. A laser beam (wave length 805 nm) irradiated LVAD out flow tube and the transmitted light or reflected scattering light was measured by an optical spectrum analyzer through an optical fiber. Measured data were processed by the signal processing technique for filtration of noise. High intensity transient signals (HITS) were simultaneously detected by TC2020 with 2.0 MHz pulsed Doppler probe. The sample volume was placed at the middle cerebral artery.
Results. Laser detected-signals correlated with HITS by TCD.

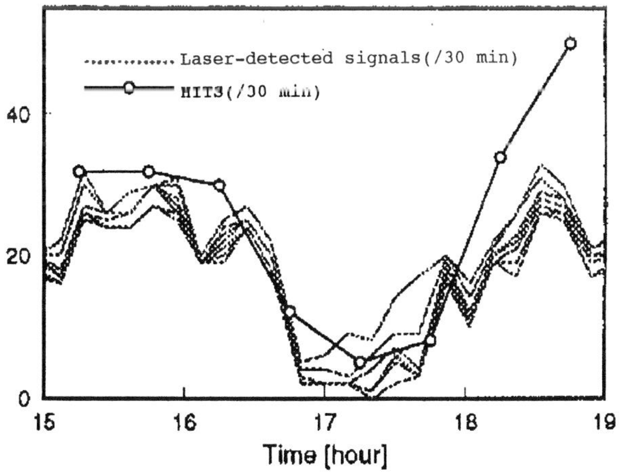

150

CAROTID RECOVERY – CASE REPORT

R.Horvath, G.Panczel, Z.Nagy
National Stroke Centre, Budapest, Hungary

Patient: We examined a 41 years old female, who collapsed three times. Her neurological examination was negative, there was substantial blood pressure difference between her arms (right: no measurable blood pressure, left: 170/90 mm Hg).
Examinations: Brain CT scan was negative. The carotid and vertebral color duplex scan showed the occlusion of the anonym artery, high grade stenosis of the left subclavian artery (SA), an intensive anterograde left vertebral artery (VA) flow, retrograde right VA flow, in the right SA distally to the origin of VA collateral anterograde flow, proximally to the origin of the VA collateral retrograde flow, in the right common carotid artery (CCA) and internal carotid artery (ICA) collateral anterograde flow. This rare circulation situation is called carotid recovery.
Operation: First dilation of the left SA, than aortic-anonym artery bypass operation were performed.
Postoperative status: During the postoperative duplex scan we found normal flows in SAs, CCAs, ICAs and VAs. Since the operation the patient is free of neurological signs and complains.

151

THE VALUE OF EXTRACRANIAL CAROTID ARTERY EXAMINATION IN BRAIN DEATH PATIENTS

D.G. Iacopino, M. Passalacqua, M. Ruggeri, C. Alafaci, F. Tomasello

Neurosurgical Clinic, University of Messina, Italy

Transcranial Doppler examination (TCD) is a non invasive method capable of detecting the interruption of cerebral flow in patients with criteria of brain death. Infact oscillating flow or systolic spikes are typical Doppler-sonographic flow signals found in the presence of cerebral circulatory arrest (CCA). In some European country this examination has been recommended by several medical councils as one of the methods able to shorten the waiting time for fulfilling the criteria for diagnosis of cerebral death. The problem is when no signal is detected. Theoretically it is impossible to say if this condition is determined by CCA detected in a later stage or by the absence of the "temporal windows".
During 1998 in our institution, a TCD study was requested in 30 patients in order to confirm CCA in brain death diagnosed patients. In one patients the TCD was negative since a diastolic, not reverberating flow was detected in the middle cerebral artery. In 11 patients (3 of them were infants < 1 y.o.) No signals were detected. In these patients an extracranial carotid artery study was performed with both the 2 MHz and 4 MHz probe. In all patients a clear reverberating flow pattern was detected confirming CCA.
In conclusion extracranial carotid artery doppler examination enhances transcranial doppler doppler sensitivity in the determination of cerebral circulatory arrest in brain death patients.

152

THE VALUE OF TCD FINDINGS IN DETECTION AND ASSESSMENT OF INTERNAL CAROTID OCCLUSIVE DISEASE

D. Jatužis, R. Mameniškienė
Department of Neurology, Vilnius University Hospital, Lithuania

Aim of the study: to evaluate the changes of intracranial circulation that could help for diagnosis and affect the clinical manifestations of internal carotid occlusive disease. **Materials and methods:** during 1995-1999 101 patients with internal carotid artery (ICA) stenoses ≥70% or occlusions were selected for the study according to the results of extracranial color-coded sonography (ECCS). Intracranial circulation was investigated by transcranial Doppler (TCD) and clinical manifestations of cerebral ischemia were recorded. The results were analysed in subgroups of patients considering the grade of ICA pathology, clinical findings, prevailing collateral circulation, vasoreactivity, and compared to the age-matched control group of persons without ICA occlusive pathology. **Results**: spontaneous intracranial collateral flow was found in 81 patients (82.7%). The prevailing collateralisation from the contralateral carotid circulation was most frequent-in 52 patients (64.2%); from the vertebrobasilar circulation-in 24 cases (29.6%); only from the external carotid artery-5 (6.2%). Pathological flow through the ophthalmic artery (OA) was present in 72 out of 100 patients (72.0%). TCD detection of any spontaneous collateral flow had sensitivity 92.9%, specificity 78.6% and accuracy 90.8% (pathological OA flow-83.1%, 92.3% and 84.8%, respectively) for ICA stenosis >80% or occlusion, compared to the conclusions of ECCS. Significant reduction of flow velocity and pulsatility index in the middle cerebral artery was confirmed on the side of pathological ICA, compared with the contralateral side and control group (t-test, p<0.001). Impaired vasoreactivity on the side of pathological ICA or bilaterally (in cases of significant bilateral ICA disease) was identified in 68.0% cases. **Conclusions**: pathological flow through the OA and spontaneous collateral flow are important diagnostic TCD markers of ICA stenosis >80% or occlusion. The most important collateral pathway is through the anterior communicating artery from the contralateral carotid circulation. Disabling cerebral ischemic events have higher incidence among the patients with impaired vasoreactivity and posterior or incomplete type of Willis' circle.

153

Transcranial Ultrasonography and Diffusion- and Perfusion-weighted MRI in eclamptic Encephalopathy

G. Jan Junge-Hülsing, K. Titus Hoffmann and Ludwig Niehaus
Department of Neurology and Department of Radiology
Charité, Virchow-Klinikum, Berlin, Germany

The pathogenesis of neurological deficits in eclampsia is still unclear. Most studies suggest that arterial hypertension in eclampsia leads to leakage of intravascular fluid causing hypertensive encephalopathy. An alternative hypothesis is that cerebral damage results from focal ischemia due to cerebral vasospasm.
We report a 29-year-old woman who developed hypertension (>190 mmHg), severe headache and a generalized seizure at 34th week of gestation. After cesaerian-section she complained of headache and blurred vision and became stuporous. Transcranial Colour Coded Sonography (TCCS) showed elevated mean blood flow velocities up to 170 cm/sec in the proximal segments of the basal cerebral arteries indicating cerebral vasospasm. Blood flow velocities within the extracranial internal carotid artery lay within the normal range excluding a hyperdynamic state of cerebral perfusion. T2-weighted and diffusion weighted MRI showed high signal lesions in left parietal and occipital lobe. These lesions were hyperintense on apparent diffusion coefficient (ADC) maps consistent with vasogenic edema. Perfusion-weighted imaging (PWI) did not reveal areas of hyper- or hypoperfusion assessed by mean time of bolus track arrival and mean transit time. The mental status and vision returned gradually to normal over approximately the next 3 days and blood pressure normalized. Follow-up TCCS examination still demonstrated pathologically elevated cerebral blood flow velocities. 8 days after delivery lesions in T2- and in DWI had completely resolved.
As shown by TCCS and PWI cerebral vasoconstriction in eclampsia is not associated with cerebral hypo- or hyperperfusion. Segmental vasospasm and vasogenic edema demonstrated by DWI may be caused by vascular endothelial damage. This case demonstrates that the combined use of TCCS and functional MRI is helpful to elucidate the pathogenesis of neurological deficits in eclampsia.

154

FUNCTIONAL TRANSCRANIAL VERTEBROBASILAR DOPPLER IN CERVICOGENIC HEADACHE

D.Kadojić*, M.Kadojić**, B.Barac*,M.Dikanović***
*Department of Neurology, University Hospital Osijek, Croatia
**Department of Physical Medicine and Rehabilitation,University Hospital Osijek,Croatia
***Department of Neurology, General Hospital Slavonski Brod,Croatia

Cervicogenic headache (CEH) is a complex syndrome characterized by deep unilateralskleletomuscular pain, autonomic reactions and a number of concomitant phenomena,with yet unclear etiopathogenesis and pathophysiology. The aim of this study was to analyze the hemodynamic changes in vertebrobasilar (VB) arteries in patients with CEH and comparison of these changes with radiological findings and neuropsychological profiles of patients.
In 1999 we diagnosed CEH in 50 out-patients of the Department of Neurology Osijek, the 42 female and 8 male, aged between 20 and 60 years (average age 44,88 years). The diagnosis was established in accordance with the criteria of Sjaastad. Functional Transcranial Doppler (TCD) of VB arteries was carried out in Neurological ultrasound laboratory with 2 MHz probe in standard position, maximum ventral and dorsal flexion, right and left rotation of head. Standard and functional cervical spine-radiographs and neuropsychological examination with Cornell index of neuroticism were performed diagnostically.
Results: Functional TCD VB was abnormal in 39 (78%), and normal in 11 (22%) patients. According to the character of the disclosed TCD changes we found signs of compressive cervical syndrome in 11 (28,2%), vasospasm in 20 (51,3%), atherosclerotic changes with a diminished flow in 4 (10.25%), and combination of atherosclerotic and compressive changes in 4 (10.25%) patients. Comparation of TCD results,radiological and neuropsychological findings showed high correlation (93,3%) between compressive TCD syndrome with degenerative changes on cervical spine (moderate 33,3%, significant 20% and heavy degenerative changes 53,3%, respectively), and high correlation (90%) between vasospasm and neuroticism (moderate grade 35% and high grade of neuroticism 55%, respectively).
Conclusion: The most of the patients with CEH had TCD abnormalities. Functional TCD VB gives clear information about character of this hemodynamic changes and is useful method in differentiating the etiopathogenetic factors and pathophysiological machanisms of CEH.

155

ULTRASOUND EVALUATION OF CEREBROVASCULAR RESERVE (CRV) WITH NITROGLYCERIN TEST.

T.V. Kaminskaya[1], M.D., T.V. Avramenco[2], M.D.
1. Diagnostic Centre, Minsk, Republic of Belarus
2. Advanced Training Institute for Doctors, Republic of Belarus.

Purpose: We wished to characterize the CVR and evaluate degree of cerebral atherosclerosis (CA) progress in prospective study.

Methods and Results: 63 patients (age 49-72, mean 62 years) with cerebrovascular disease were investigated with transcranial dopler (TCD) – sonography with using of sublingual-functional nitroglycerin test (0,25 mg). The subjects were divided into three groups according to their changes of TCD-circulation after nitroglycerin test. There were: adequate, paradoxal and negative reaction.

In prospective study during 36-month period we founded:

1) The stable character CA with adequate pharmacologyc reaction was observed in 36% of subjects; in 13% cases was the change from paradoxal and negative to adequate; in 35% – was founded the progress of CA with increasing the dopplerografic deficities blood flows and changing reactions from adequate to negative
2) The best results indicated stabilization of CA were founded in regular treatment patients (with antiaggregates, hypotensive, hypocholesterole drugs)

Conclusion: TCD with the nitroglycerin test is simple to perform and high-sensitive evaluation of cerebrovascular dynamics in patients with CA.

156

STROKE SYMPTOMATIC AS A FIRST SYMPTOM IN-PATIENTS WITH MULTIPLE SCLEROSIS (MS)

D.KOUNTOURIS
Center For Neurological Diagnosis, Michalakopoulou 45, 11528, Athens, Hellas

In a group of 1258 MS patients, 361 males and 897 females aged 47 ± 2,5 years and with length of illness 9,5 ± 3,1 years, examined in a ten year period. In 12 of these patients seven presented symptoms of transitory ischemic attack and the remaining five reported typical hemiparesis and hemepisthesia similar to one caused by stroke. 9 of the 12 patients were 25 to 35 years old and the rest were over 40.
All patients were suspected of having suffered typical vascular disturbances and only after throughout studies was it found that they were suffering from MS. This diagnosis was accomplished through repeated neurological examinations, MRI and labor chemical examination. What was significant was that in-patients the typical examinations, in their entirety, for the establishment of the presence of MS was not pathological. The findings in more recent tests showed some pathological results. It is noteworthy that all patients have maintained a very good condition and particularly those that received in the early stage of the disease immunosuppressive and immumodulated treatment.
Conclusion: Stroke symptomatology especially temporary one might be beginning of MS. This should be treated as a possibility of alternative diagnosis. Especially in such case early diagnosis and proper treatment contributes greatly to a good prognosis.

157

Detection of multifocal deep intracerebral microbleedings using T_2*-gradient-echo-MRI is related to hypertensive microangiopathy

C. Kukla[1], HR. Siebner[1], K. Winbeck[1], Th. Wilhelm[2], H. Gräfin von Einsiedel[2], B. Conrad[1], D. Sander[1]

Department of [1]Neurology and [2]Neuroradiology, Technical University of Munich, Germany

Background:
T_2*-weighted gradient-echo magnetic resonance imaging (MRI) is considered to be useful in the detection of intracerebral hemosiderin deposits due to old hemorrhages.
Patients:
We report on 5 patients with gait disorder, hyperreflexia, and cognitive impairment. All patients showed multifocal hypointense cerebral lesions (>5) in T_2* -gradient-echo MRI due to chronic microbleedings, which were mainly located in the brainstem, basal ganglia and cerebellum. Associated MRI findings were widespread leukoaraiosis and lacunar infarcts. All patients had a history of severe arterial hypertension, 4 patients presented with slight elevated levels of blood pressure in the 24h blood pressure recordings.
Discussion:
The clinical and MRI data of the presented patients suggest that arterial hypertension plays a important role in the development of microbleedings in the deep cerebral structures. Further investigation is necessary to reveal possible relationships with amyloid angiopathy and Alzheimer's disease.

158

CRITERIAL OF INTRACRANIAL STENOSES WITH TRANSCRANIAL COLOR DOPPLER

Malferrari G. , Guidetti D.Zucco R.,Pisanello A., Marcello N., Accorsi . *, Moratto R.**, Coppi G. **, Ragazzi G. **,Galletti G.***, Sanguignl S.°, Curatola C.°, Landini G.P.°°, Meneghetti G.°°°. Baracchini C..Manara R.°°° , Prati P §. , Zanette E. Neurology Dept Reggio Emilia , S.Maria Nuova;*Angiology Dept Bologna, Ospedale Maggiore;**Vascular Surgery Dept ,Modena Ospedale Civile ;***Neurology Dept Forli , Ospedale Civile "Neurology Department San Benedetto del Tronto ; °° Medicine Dept Firenze . °°° Neurology Dept University of Padova ,[1]. Neurophisiology Service Udine,Neurology Dept Roma .
Currently there is not an established criteria for intracranial arterial stenoses. However from January 1998 to August 1999, 119 articles appeared in literature about this problem. From the Ringelstain criteria we have moved on to the most recent study of Wong (1998) and Baumgarten (1999);in our experience we think that the evaluation of intracranial stenoses should be made in the first, with transcranial Color coded duplex sonography for diverse problems: the angle of correction and the use of enhanced contrast medium. Our criteria for validation of intracranial stenoses are in agreement with Baumgarten in particular for the MCA > 120 cm./sec. (peak systolic); beside this we consider the difference in the peak systolic between opposite arteries (>50 %). From January 1999 to now we have studied 658 patients with TCCS. 126 have presented acute stroke and we have detect the presence of intracranial stenoses (IS) in 57 patients. Finally in the other patients in particular in which they have an extracranial stenoses was found in 30%. For these purpose we are presently conducting an on-going pluricentric study regarding these problems, comparing the different diagnostic methods such as Angio-RM, Angio CT scan and ECTCD

159

ULTRASOUND EVALUATION OF ATHEROSCLEROSIS AND INTRACRANIAL CIRCULATION IN PATIENTS WITH DEMENTIA

R. Mameniškienė, D. Jatužis, G. Kaubrys
Department of Neurology, Vilnius University Hospital, Lithuania

Aim of the study: to evaluate the association of atherosclerosis and changes of intracranial circulation with Alzheimer's disease and vascular dementia. **Materials and methods:** consecutive patients with probable Alzheimer's disease (AD), vascular dementia (VaD) and age-matched control subjects were selected for the study. Extracranial and intracranial cerebral arteries were evaluated by color-coded duplex sonography and transcranial Doppler. Indicators of atherosclerosis included intima-media thickness (IMT), plaques of the carotid arteries and ankle-to-brachial systolic blood pressure ratio. Based on these indicators participants were dichotomized as mild/no atherosclerosis (0 or 1 indicators positive) and moderate/severe atherosclerosis (2 or 3 indicators positive). Intracranial flow velocities, pulsatility indices (PI) and transient hyperemic response ratio (THRR), as a measure of vasoreactivity, were calculated and compared between the groups. **Results**: 66 patients were investigated up-to-date (mean±SD): 1) AD group-n=32, age 73.5±7.0 yrs; 2) VaD group-n=16, age 67.1±8.1 yrs; 3) control group-n=18, age 71.1±8.1 yrs. Trend to have higher atherosclerosis scores was found in VaD group compared to control group (Fisher exact test, p=.072) but not in AD group (p=.384). No significant difference was found between AD and VaD groups according to atherosclerosis score. IMT in VaD group was significantly higher compared to AD and control groups (mean IMT mm±SD in VaD group-1.14±.20; AD-.99±.21; control group-.90±.14; t-test p=.0003 and p=.023). MCA PI was higher in both dementia groups, but it did not reach statistical significance: PI in VaD group-1.16±.23; AD group-1.12±.20; control group-1.05±.20. Significantly lower cerebral vasoreactivity was found in VaD patients compared to other groups. **Conclusions**: atherosclerosis score has a trend to be higher in patients with vascular dementia. Association of atherosclerosis with Alzheimer's disease is not clear from available data. Increased intracranial resistance to blood flow in both dementia groups might reflect higher incidence of microangiopathy.

160

CERVICAL ARTERIO-VENOUS FISTULAS – ULTRASONOGRAPHIC CONSIDERATIONS

D. Marinescu, C. Tiu, O. Bajenaru
- DEPARTMENT OF NEUROLOGY -
UNIVERSITY HOSPITAL – BUCHAREST ROMANIA

We present our experience of 6 cases of arterio-venous fistulas in the basal cervical region. These are rare vascular malformations between the common carotid or the subclavian artery and the jugular vein. 2 of the cases recognised a local trauma in the past, but in 4 cases no trauma or other obvious cause could be identified. They become clinically manifest as pulsatile, depressible, enlarging over time masses at the base of the neck, with vascular murmurs over them. 3 of them were not noticed by patients and were incidentally diagnosed during a standard Doppler examination for an unrelated simptomatology. The ultrasonographic examination revealed high local arterial velocities and a markedly dilated jugular vein with significantly increased, turbulent local flow and abnormally accelerated flap of the venous valves. The duplex colour-coded examination revealed the arterio-venous communication in 5 cases. All cases had digital substraction angiography which confirmed diagnosis. We discuss the pathophysiological mechanisms involved and we assess the contribution of ultrasonography for diagnosis and management of these patients.

161

Neurosonology in the Follow-up of Patients After Carotid Endarterectomy

L.Németh[1], Cs Grósz[1], L Tarsoly[2], Zs.Varga[3], J.Nikl[1]
County Hosp.Zalaegerszeg, Dept .of Neurology,Surgery[2] and Cardiosurgery[3],Hungary

Introduction: The authors investigated the role of cervical duplex sonography in taking care of the patients who underwent carotid endarterectomy. They searched for the most frequent changes causing complications, and for differences between the operation methods considering the long-term prognosis.

Methods and results: The first duplex ultrasonography was usually made one month after the operation, and 3 and 6 months later it was repeated. Then the development of the restenosis on the operated part, changes in the Doppler spectrum and the velocity of flow, the neointima-media thickness, and the existence of a possible intima stair were investigated. They evaluated the material of 54 patients. The average age of life was 65,8 years the follow-up time was performed 37,8 months. 4 patients had bilateral operations. Eversion endarterectomies (EEA) were performed in 27 cases, conventional thrombendarterectomies (TEA) in 31 cases (3 times with patch plastics).. 52 patients received antiplatelet therapy permanently, 40 of them received aspirin, and 12 ticlopidine. 2 patients were given cumerine. The most important risk factors were hypertension (in 34 cases) and hypercholesterinemy (in 30 cases).

The velocity of blood flow normalised right after the operation, the Doppler spectrum and the structure of the vessel wall normalised usually after 3 months. Permanent vessel wall thickenings were observed in 21 cases (36%) and turbulent flows (color methods) in 24 cases (41%). The retrograde ophthalmic arterial circulation and the middle cerebral arterial flow normalised in all of the cases. There was no stroke death. After EEA 1 early restenosis free of complaints, 1 permanent distal intima step, 11 vessel wall thickenings (41%) were found. After TEA a 25% restenosis was observed in 1 case, a late reocclusion free of complaints and permanent distal intima step was found in 1 case, wall thickenings in the operated area were observed in 13 cases (42%) Recidive stroke on the operated side after the perioperative period was not observed. Minor strokes of the other vessel areas were found in the cases of 5 patients. The unoperated carotid arterial side showed 6 times vessel wall sclerosis, 29 times low grade, 8 times middle grade stenosis, and 3 times carotid occlusion.

Conclusions: In this material the development of late restenosis and neurologic complications was not influenced by the fact of the type of the operation. The number of the restenoses is minimal, significant restenosis was not found. During the follow-up examinations you have to search for "minor symptoms" like neointima- media thickening and turbulence, which occur frequently. You have to pay big attention to the status of the other supraortic vessel, the level of serum cholesterol, blood pressure, the psychical status, that means complex check-ups are necessary.

162

DISSECTION OF THE CRANIOCERVICAL ARTERIES

M.Bošnjak Pašić, V.Demarin, V.Vargek Solter, T.Breitenfeld, H.Hećimović

University Department of Neurology, "Sestre milosrdnice" University Hospital, Vinogradska 29, Zagreb, Croatia

Dissections of the craniocervical arteries (carotid and vertebral) are acute disruptions of the arterial wall. They are a relatively uncommon cause of stroke in general populatic . out more commonly are the cause of stroke in younger patients, parti .rly women. Dissections are generally divided into two groups: spon ,us and traumatic. Often multivessel dissections can be seen.

We have investigated 8 patients (4 men and 4 women) age 41 to 66 years, with a dissection of the carotid or vertebral artery. Clinical presentation, ultrasonographic examination (transcranial color Doppler and color coded duplex sonography of carotid and vertebral arteries) and neuroimaging (CT and DSA) were followed up.

Dissections were spontaneous in 6 patients and posttraumatic in 2 cases. Common clinical manifestations included headache, pain in the neck and focal cerebral symptoms. Seven patients were hypertensive, 3 had hyperlipoproteinaemia and 2 were diabetics. Five patients had the dissection of the internal carotid artery, 2 of the vertebral artery and one patient had ipsilateral dissection of the carotid and vertebral artery. One patient with the dissection of the internal artery also had an intracranial aneurysm. Two patients were treated operatively, 5 with anticoagulation therapy and one with antithrombotic therapy. In follow up after received therapy, 6 patients had partial clinical improvement and improvement in ultrasonographic findings in the dissected arteries. One patient had stroke after surgery with deterioration of neurological deficit. One patient which was treated only with antithrombotic therapy, after 3 months had recurrent fatal stroke.

Early clinical, noninvasive ultrasound and radiological detection of craniocervical artery dissection is necessary. Immediate anticoagulation therapy must be introduced in order to minimize morbidity and mortality due to this condition.

163

SPEED ASYMMETRY IN BILATERAL VMCA HAS A BENIGN INFLUENCE ON VELOCITY CHANGES WHILE THINKING

A. E. Roberts, Neurosonology Research Laboratory, Department of Psychology, Catawba College, Salisbury NC USA

BACKGROUND. Many persons show natural hemisphere asymmetry in blood flow velocity. This asymmetry might affect the degrees of change in velocity induced by a cortical activation procedure. We studied this possibility using transcranial Doppler (TCD) sonography to obtain simultaneous bilateral velocity measures in the middle cerebral artery (VMCA) during sets of thinking activities. METHODS. Men and women college students served in a 2 X 5 repeated-measures factorial design. VMCA rate (fast vs slow, regardless of hemisphere) and experimental phases were the factors. A 31-sec, eyes-closed baseline (BL) was followed by four, 31-sec thinking tasks: brief remembering, creating a personal image, constructing new words from the letters of a target word, and solving a simple math problem. RESULTS. Of our 72 subjects, 54 showed hemisphere asymmetry in VMCA: a mean VMCA from one side was outside the range of measures calculated for the other (mean VMCA +/- 1 SD). VMCA in the right hemisphere was faster for 23 subjects and was faster for 31 in the left. Speed asymmetry was not related to gender or handedness. VMCA in the "faster" side was about 15% more than in the "slower" side. VMCA accelerated bilaterally over VBL during the four thinking tasks, but the degrees of change (ranges: 4.0%-to-6.8%) were not related to speed asymmetry. CONCLUSIONS. The presence of hemisphere asymmetry in bilateral VMCA does not affect the degrees of change in VMCA when induced by a cortical activation procedure using thinking tasks.

164

RESTENOSIS AFTER ANGIOPLASTY AND STENTING OF THE CAROTID BIFURCATION

I. Saïd [1], M.C.C. van der Mee [1], E.S. Louwerse [1], J.M.P.G. Ernst [2], H.W. Mauser [3], T.Th.C. Overtoom [4], J.C. van den Berg [4], R.G.A. Ackerstaff [1].
From the departments of Clinical Neurophysiology [1], Cardiology [2], Neurology [3] en Radiology [4].
Vascular Centre, St. Antonius Hospital Nieuwegein, the Netherlands.

Introduction: Percutaneous transluminal angioplasty and stenting is recently used as a method to treat carotid stenosis. It has the potential adventage of being an endovascular approach, requires no surgical incision or general anaesthesia and may result in a shorter hospital stay and lower health care costs. In order to find out whether this method, with respect to restenosis, is a alternative for carotid endarterectomy (CEA) we performed carotid artery duplex scanning in 100 patients during follow-up.
Methods: Between november 1997 and november 1999 we examined 100 patients with high grade carotid stenosis who underwent carotid angioplasty and stenting (CAS). In all patients a duplex examination was performed one day before and one day after the intervention and a follow-up 3, 12 and 24 months there after.
Results: All patients had a duplex one day after CAS. Until now, 84% of the patients had a duplex scan at 3 months and 33% at one year after the intervention. One day after the procedure, only one patient had a haemodynamically significant (≥65%) residual stenosis. At 3 months we observed a ≥65% stenosis in 7 patients (8%), and at one year in 5 patients (15%). The majority of the 12 patients with a significant stenosis at 3 and 12 months also had a 50- 65% stenosis at day one.
In a follow-up study of 109 patients who underwent CEA in our hospital the rate of ≥65% restenosis at 3 and 12 months are 2% and 4%, respectively.
Conclusion: Residual stenosis and early restenosis during the first year after CAS occur in a substantial number of patients. So far, the rate of restenosis after CAS significantly exceeds our experience with restenosis after CEA. However, further follow-up studies are required.

165

STRUCTURAL CHANGES OF THE INSULAR CORTEX IN ESSENTIAL ARTERIAL HYPERTENSION DEMONSTRATED WITH VOXEL-BASED MRI MORPHOMETRY

D. Sander, K. Winbeck, J. Klingelhöfer*, H. Poppert, J. Schwarze*, B. Conrad
Dept. of Neurology, Technical University of Munich and *Klinikum Chemnitz, Germany

Increasing evidence links essential arterial hypertension to an increased sympathetic activity. Interestingly several experimental and clinical studies demonstrated an important role of the insular cortex in the cortical control of the regulation of the sympathetic nervous system.
In the present study we evaluated 38 patients with essential hypertension compared to 37 normotensive age- and sex-matched controls using MRI voxel-based morphometry to search for subtle cerebral morphological differences between both groups, particularly in the insula region. All patients underwent MR imaging with T1-weighted scans (3d-turbo FLASH sequence, voxel-volume 1x1x1.5 mm). Voxel-based morphometry (Wright et al., Neuroimage 1995) involved spatial normalisation according to Talairach and Tournoux, segmenting of grey matter, correcting for volume changes, isotropic gaussian filtering and, finally, doing a statistical analysis to localize differences between groups. The final voxel-based group comparison revealed several regions with significant structural differences in grey matter density between both groups. However, after correction for multiple comparisons we observed a significant difference only for the insular cortex, in particular the anterior part (Talairach coordinates x=+10, y=-8, z=37; Z-Score=4.02; p<0.001). This difference consisted of an decrease in volume of the anterior insular cortex and a reduced density of the grey matter in this region in the group with essential hypertension.
Our findings indicate subtle structural changes of the insular cortex in essential arterial hypertension with a decreased neuronal density in this region that cannot be detected by conventional MRI. Our data point to a possible role of the insular cortex in the pathogenesis of essential arterial hypertension.

166

Echodensity of carotid plaques, cerebral Embolus Signals (ES) and collateral circulation during Carotid Endarterectomy (CE).

V.A.Shakhnovich, V.A.Lazarev, G.E.Mitroshin, M.V.Churilov, D.Y.Usachev, A.A.Shmigelsky, A.Y.Lubnin
Burdenko Neurosurgery Institute, Moscow, Russia.

Aim: To study echodensity of carotid plaques, ES and collateral circulation during CE.
Material and methods: Perioperative monitoring of FV in both MCA's was performed in 30 pts with symptomatic carotid stenosis (m 36, age 46-67y) having undergone a total CE due to stenosis of ICA of 50-95%. The contralateral ICA was normal in 21 pts, stenosed/occluded in 11/7 pts. Extracranial and transcranial Color Coded Duplex was used to assess the size of carotid plaques and patency of Circle of Willis. The perantage reduction of FV (PRFV) in MCA on TCD during clamping ICA upon CE measured reserve capacity of collateral circulation, caused mainly by the state of Circle of Willis, contralateral ICA and VA. All images of plaques were standardized using a linear scaling with two reference points so that gray scale median (GSM) of blood was 7 and of adventitia 70 on a scale of 0-225 (0 - black, 225 - white). GSM of plaque measured its echodensity: GSM ≤ 15 - echolucent plaque (ELP), GSM > 15 - echogenic plaque (EGP). Bilateral TCD monitorings of MCAs were performed for 1 h. to assess ES according to internationally accepted definition.
Results: Combination of disturbances of Circle of Willis with stenosis/occlusion of contralateral ICA led usually to increase of PRFV (more than 50%). ES were significantly (p<0.001) more frequent (16 +/- 4 in 1 hour) in ELP than EGP. (3 +/- in 1 hour). It was established in ELP the same frequency of small and high PRFV (less and more than 50%) suggesting an embolic pathogenesis of stroke. On the other hand in EGP high PRFV (>50%) happened significantly more often (p<0.001) than in small PRFV (≤50%) suggesting a haemodynamic pathogenesis of stroke.
Conclusion: ELP are characterized mainly by an embolic but EGP - mainly by haemodynamic pathogenesis of stroke.

167

PECULIARITIES IN REGIONAL CEREBRAL BLOOD FLOW OF TERM AND PRETERM INFANTS

A.Sugak, I.Dvoryakovsky, G.Yatsyk
Department of Radiology, Research Center of Child Health, Moscow, Russia

To evaluate the peculiarities in regional cerebral blood flow (CBF) of term and preterm infants we investigated CBF velocities in anterior cerebral (ACA), internal carotid (ICA) and basilar (BA) arteries by color Doppler imaging in 45 term and 58 preterm infants during the first three months of life.

Arterial velocities increased significantly (p<0,01) with the increase of body weight, gestational and postnatal age. However, intensiveness of this process in different arteries was dissimilar in term and preterm infants. In term infants proportional increase of CBF velocities took place in all arteries without regional differences during first three months of life. In preterm infants correlation coefficients between body weight and postnatal age on one hand and minimal and mean CBF velocíties in ACA and BA on the other hand were significantly higher (p<0,05) than in ICA. It means that CBF velocities in ACA and BA increased more intensive than in ICA, especially in infants with gestational age less than 34 weeks.

Our study demonstrates in vivo a heterochrony of nervous receptors system formation in various cerebral arteries. The morphologists determined that middle cerebral artery as a continuation of ICA had the highest concentration of nervous fibres in vascular walls because development of MCA wall structures leaves other cerebral arteries behind.

168

PATENT FORAMEN OVALE, MIGRAINE AND STROKE: A POSSIBLE LINK ?

R Sztajzel*, S Roth, D Genoud, J Le Floch-Rohr,*
Department of Neurology (Prof T Landis) and Neurosonology Unit*
University Hospital Geneva, Switzerland

Recent studies have reported an increased prevalence of PFO in patients with migraine with aura. To investigate the possible relationship between migraine with aura and paradoxical embolism, we studied the prevalence and characteristics of both conditions in 65 patients presenting an acute stroke or TIA. The patients were questioned about migraine with or without aura according to the criteria of the International Headache Society. PFO was found in 37 of 65 patients. Thirteen of these 37 patients with PFO (35%) had a history of migraine with aura as compared to 3 (11 %) of the 28 patients without PFO ($X2 = 4.8$ $p < 0.05$). In 19 patients in whom the PFO was considered to play a causal role for stroke, 10 (53%) had a history of migraine with aura ($X2 = 1.6$, $p = 0.95$) whereas in 14 patients, in whom PFO was considered unrelated, only 2 (14%) patients had a migraine with aura. In 4 patients the responsibility of the PFO could not be determined. Migraineurs with PFO were likely to experience a migraine-like episode at the onset of the vascular event while not the migraineurs without PFO ($X2 = 8.7$, $p < 0.01$).
Conclusion : Prevalence of migraine with aura is high among stroke-patients with PFO. In patients with a high presumption of paradoxical embolism, the proportion of migraineurs with aura is increased and suggests a possible role of this association in the occurrence of the cerebrovascular event.

169

Multiple intracranial aneurysms in fibromuscular dysplasia associated with a tight embolizing intracranial carotid artery stenosis

W. Weger[1], G.E. Klein[2], M. Duft[1], S. Horner[1], K. Niederkorn[1]
Departments of Neurology[1] and Radiology[2], Karl-Franzens-University, Graz, Austria

Fibromuscular dysplasia is an uncommon idiopathic, systemic vascular disease also involving the intracranial vessels and often presenting as a transient ischemic attack, stroke or as a subarachnoid hemorrhage because of its association with intracranial aneurysms.
We report a 39-year old female patient who was admitted because of paresthesias and a severe headache. At the age of 36 she suffered a subarachnoid hemorrhage due to aneurysmal rupture.
Transcranial Doppler sonography showed an increase of the blood flow velocity in the leftsided C-1 segment (maximum mean flow velocity 142 cm/sec). The findings on lumbar puncture were unremarkable.
Four-vessel-angiography disclosed a hypoplastic A-1 segment and a narrowing of the leftsided C-1 segment in front of two aneurysms.
Hyperintensive transient signals (HITS) suggesting embolism originating from the stenosis were detected during TCD-monitoring.
Implantation of Gugeliemi detachable coils and percutaneous transluminal angioplasty were performed. Blood flow velocity decreased and no further HITS were detectable by TCD-monitoring. Clinical outcome was good.

170

OPHTHALMIC ARTERY EVALUATION IN RETINAL AND OPTIC NERVE ISCHEMIA OR EMBOLISM

Christine Wijman, Ira Galin, Val Pochay, Michael Winter, Behrooz Koleini, Ippolit Matjucha, Viken Babikian. Boston University School of Medicine, Boston, MA

Purpose: To assess ophthalmic artery (OA) hemodynamic changes as they relate to retinal and optic nerve arterial occlusive disease. **Methods:** Consecutive patients with retinal or optic nerve ischemia or embolism referred to the Ophthalmology and Neurology Departments over a 22 month period were screened. Eighty-four satisfied selection criteria, and 72 (mean age 68.6 years, 78 affected eyes), had technically satisfactory TCD studies of the ophthalmic arteries. All underwent cardiac, cerebrovascular, and hematological evaluations. Controls were obtained by reviewing the Neurovascular Laboratory's records of 100 consecutive patients, and 23 individuals (mean age 65.3 years, 40 control eyes) with magnetic resonance angiography or duplex ultrasound evidence of bilateral less than 50% internal carotid artery stenosis were selected. TCD testing was performed on TC-2020 instruments. In an effort to avoid contamination from flow in the ipsilateral internal carotid artery siphon and middle and anterior cerebral arteries, each OA was insonated at a depth of 45 to 55 mm. **Results:** For the control group, mean and standard deviation values for OA peak systolic flow velocities were 38.2 +/- 11.4 cm/sec at 45 mm, 38.4 +/- 10.0 cm/sec at 50 mm, and 39.9 +/- 10.0 cm/sec at 55 mm. In the patient group, flow velocities exceeded the control mean + 2 standard deviation values in 5 patients (6.9%), 1 with optic nerve infarction, 2 with retinal infarction, and 2 with asymptomatic retinal embolism. OA flow was retrograde in 5 (6.9%) patients but in no controls. Two of these patients had optic nerve infarction and 3 had transient monocular blindness. Five of 16 (31.3%) patients with retinal or optic nerve infarction and 5 of 57 (8.8%) patients with transient monocular blindness or asymptomatic retinal embolism had either increased velocities or retrograde flow ($p=0.035$). **Conclusion:** In patients with retinal embolism or ischemia, markedly increased flow velocities indicative of ophthalmic artery stenosis are uncommon. Hemodynamic changes are detected in 13.7% of cases and are relatively more common in those with optic nerve or retinal infarction. TCD testing may be useful in assessing some patients with retinal and optic nerve arterial occlusive disease.

171

Decoupling of cerebral perfusion and glucose metabolism in eclampsia

P. Zunker[1], A.L. Georgiadis[1], Norbert Czech[2], Johann Steffens[3], Kerstin Golombeck[4], Günther Deuschl[1] Departments of Neurology [1], Nuclear Medicine [2], Diagnostic Radiology [3], and Gynaecology [4], Kiel University Hospital, Niemannsweg 147, 24105 Kiel, Germany

The pathophysology underlying the reversible neurologic manifestation in eclampsia is still open. We report on a 34 year old woman with eclampsia who was repetitively examined by transcranial Doppler (TCD), magnetic resonance imaging (MRI), i.e. T1- and T2-weighted images, perfusion measurements and magnetic resonance angiography (MRA), and ^{18}F-fluoro-2-deoxy-D-glucose positron emission tomography (FDG-PET).

During the acute phase, transcranial ultrasound showed elevated flow velocities bilaterally in the anterior, middle and posterior cerebral arteries as well as in the internal carotid arteries. Repetitive MRA was without any signs for vasospasm and MRI perfusion measurements showed completely homogeneous cerebral blood flow. In the initial phase T2-weighted images revealed predominantly bilateral frontal and parietal hyperintesities. FDG-PET showed inhomogeneous glucose metabolism with primary increased glucose utilisation in these hyperintens T2-weighted areas. TCD, MRI, and PET examinations after 3 weeks were normal.

These findings support the concept of vasodilatation with consecutive hyperperfusion and vasogenic oedema due to a damage of the blood-brain barrier in eclamptic women. Additionally, they show for the first time that in the presence of homogenous perfusion mainly glucose metabolism is increased, suggesting a decoupling of cerebral perfusion and glucose metabolism in eclampsia. The elevated glucose metabolism might indicate an increased neuronal activity in women with eclampsia.

Cerebrovascular Diseases

Author Index

Numbers refer to Abstract No.

Fax + 41 61 306 12 34
E-Mail karger@karger.ch
www.karger.com

© 2000 S. Karger AG, Basel

MAIN SPONSORS

BRACCO
DWL
GE-ULTRASOUND
MALLINCKRODT
NICOLET-EME
SCHERING

SPONSORS

BAYER
BOEHRINGER INGELHEIM
CODMAN/DEPUY
KNOLL AG
KWIZDA
LANNACHER
NOVARTIS
NYCOMED AUSTRIA
SANOFI WINTHROP

EXHIBITORS

ACUSON
AGILENT
DWL
GE-ULTRASOUND
NICOLET-EME
SIEMENS
SCHERING
SPENCER TECHNOLOGIES
TOSHIBA